Finding ways to cope with bladder illness is often a slow, painful and bewildering experience. Bladder Health UK provides information and support to anyone suffering from chronic bladder illness and welcomes this comprehensive and engaging book which is suitable for both the sufferer and the medical professional.

Bladder Health UK

Dedications

Megan would like to dedicate this book to her best friend Tessa Lacey. Tess, I hope you know how much you mean to me – your support over the years has kept me going, especially during the wedding planning! I don't really know what I'd do without you, bestie, and I thank the moon and stars every day that you landed in my life. Love ya.

Christine would like to dedicate this book to all the fantastic people in Pop Chorus Suffolk, especially her two adoptive sisters Donna Wiles and Linda Perkins. Thanks to both of you for everything we've shared; 2016–2017 has been amazing, the best, and I look forward to all the great experiences yet to come. I love you lots!!

What's Up With Your Bladder?

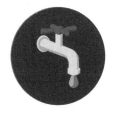

Dr Megan A Arroll and
Professor Christine P Dancey

With a Foreword by Elaine Miller

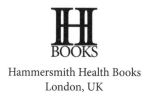

Hammersmith Health Books
London, UK

First published in 2018 by Hammersmith Health Books – an imprint of
Hammersmith Books Limited
4/4A Bloomsbury Square, London WC1A 2RP, UK
www.hammersmithbooks.co.uk

Disclaimer: The information contained in this book is for educational purposes
only. It is the result of the study and experience of the authors. Whilst the
information and advice offered are believed to be true and accurate at the
time of going to press, neither the authors nor the publisher can accept any
legal responsibility or liability for any errors or omissions that may have been
made for any adverse effects which may occur as a result of following the
recommendations given herein. Always consult a qualified medical practitioner
if you have any concerns regarding your health.

British Library Cataloguing in Publication Data: A CIP record of this book is
available from the British Library.

Print ISBN 978-1-78161-102-9
Ebook ISBN 978-1-78161-103-6

Commissioning editor: Georgina Bentliff
Designed and typeset by: Julie Bennett, Bespoke Publishing Ltd
Cover design by: Sylvia Kwan
Index: Dr Laurence Errington
Production: Helen Whitehorn, Path Projects Ltd
Printed and bound by: TJ International Ltd

Contents

About the authors

Dr Megan Arroll (PhD, CPsychol, CSci, FHEA, AFBPsS) is a psychologist who specialises in stress and anxiety, invisible/misunderstood illness and integrative approaches to healthcare. Megan has held academic positions at a number of universities and lectures on a range of topics, including mental health, the psychology of health & illness and research methods. Over recent years Megan has been writing books for patients, their families and people working with long-term conditions as well as working with individuals and organisations to improve health. To date she has published four books including *Chronic Fatigue Syndrome: What You Need to Know About CFS/ME* (SPCK), *The Menopause Maze: The Complete Guide to Conventional, Complementary and Self-Help Options* (Singing Dragon) with Liz Efiong and *Irritable Bowel Syndrome: navigating your way to recovery* with Christine Dancey.

Professor Christine Dancey (PhD, CPsychol., CHealth Psychol, FHEA, FBPsS) is Professor Emeritus of Chronic Illness Research at the University of East London (UEL) and best-selling author. Her numerous titles include *Statistics Without Maths for Psychology* (Pearson) which has been used to help many thousands of students understand the complex mathematics involved in scientific research. Christine was also the joint founder of the IBS Network and its publication *Gut Reaction* (www.theibsnetwork. org/gut-reaction/), which is now available as an online download for members. As a researcher into invisible long-term conditions and a misdiagnosed sufferer from IBS symptoms (she actually had endometriosis), she has a unique insight into what people with invisible illnesses and their families and friends want and need to know.

Megan met Christine at the University of East London, where Christine led the Chronic Illness Research Team. Within this research group, Megan and Christine published numerous papers on long-term conditions such as CFS/ME, Ménière's disease and irritable bowel syndrome (IBS). When the pair's students started to ask for easy-to-read books about some of these illnesses, Megan and Christine decided to start writing for the general public. Their first title was *Invisible Illness: Coping with Misunderstood Conditions* (SPCK), followed by *Irritable Bowel Syndrome: Navigating Your Way to Recovery* (Hammersmith Health Books). These books, together with *What's Up With Your Bladder?* include the very latest scientific research to keep patients up to date with developments in treatments and potential causes of ill health, in addition to practical advice on how to manage symptoms. Megan and Christine's shared personal experience of invisible illness has given them not only the basis for a fulfilling writing partnership, but also a deep friendship.

Acknowledgements

We would like to thank Bladder Health UK, firstly for all the wonderful work they do in this area, and secondly for permitting us to include some of their material in this book. We thank the charity also for their kind words regarding our work.

We would also like to thank Elaine Miller who fitted us into her tremendously busy schedule while she was on her sell-out Edinburgh Fringe run of shows. Your vast knowledge and unique take on all things down below was not only insightful but refreshing!

Next, we would like to thank Jo Johnstone, as always, for her expert proof-reading and feedback. We would also like to thank Sophia Woodward, who carefully read our manuscript and provided detailed feedback – the book has benefited from her suggestions.

Finally, we would also like to thank all the people with bladder conditions who kindly gave their time to share their personal experiences of bladder problems and who gave permission to use their narratives in the book.

Preface

What's Up With Your Bladder? is the third book Megan and Christine have worked on together and Christine says the last!

We came to writing books for patients following our own health issues. We've documented these experiences in our other books (see *IBS: Navigating Your Way to Recovery* also published by Hammersmith Health Books) but as health (and illness unfortunately, for some) is a lifelong journey, things have changed since the IBS book was published. Megan was diagnosed in August of 2016 with Elhers Danlos syndrome (hypermobility type, also called Type 3) which accounts for the seemingly random constellations of symptoms she's experienced for a quarter of a century, including bladder symptoms.

In *What's Up With Your Bladder?*, we've focused on the most common bladder issues, such as stress incontinence and overactive bladder syndrome, but we've also included a chapter on bladder cancer as many of us fear cancer when we have bodily symptoms. However, bladder cancer is relatively rare and the incidence is decreasing (most likely due to the drop in numbers of people smoking).

Overall, bladder symptoms are very frequent – if you've never experienced bladder trouble it's likely that you know someone who has or does, even if they don't talk about it. There is still a great deal of stigma attached to incontinence and this is why we thought it so important to talk about this hidden problem that so many people suffer from in silence. We hope by doing so, readers will be encouraged to seek help and recover their health.

Foreword

Of all the thing that people find difficult to talk about, incontinence is always discussed in hushed tones. People manage their symptoms alone, often for years, instead of speaking to their GP. I think that's often because of a belief that incontinence cannot be helped, which is a myth. Most people can improve, if not resolve, their bladder's impact on their day-to-day lives. That is why I am pleased to see Dr Arroll and Prof Dancey's book. They make the anatomy, function and evidence-based advice so clear that I am confident that reading this book will improve your bladder health.

Elaine Miller, physiotherapist and stand-up comedian

www.gussetgrippers.co.uk

How to use this book

You may already have a diagnosis of one of the conditions covered in this book. In that case you may want to go ahead and turn to the relevant chapter, but we would encourage you to read Chapter 1 also as this is a general introduction.

The book then goes onto explain in brief the anatomy of the urinary system (Chapter 2) and how the bladder and brain communicate (Chapter 3). We've included this information as it can be helpful for us to know how our bodies work, and what can go wrong, when coming to terms with an illness. Having some knowledge of these concepts can also make it easier to talk to doctors about symptoms and understand why they're suggesting a particular treatment. Developing a good relationship with your GP or specialist can help in many ways – it can be empowering to have knowledge of our condition, make it easier to discuss somewhat embarrassing symptoms and share the burden of ill health.

The next chapter of the book (Chapter 4) covers an area we are very interested in – the microbiota. Scientists, researchers and medical doctors now appreciate the importance of the various micro-organisms which live in our guts. Our gut microbiota keep us healthy. If they get out of balance, our health can deteriorate. Disturbances in the microbiota are associated with IBS and other conditions, which may include bladder problems. This chapter helps you understand what you can do in order to maintain a healthy diversity of microbiota.

Then, Chapters 5 to 7 look at individual bladder conditions, including interstitial cystitis, and the associated symptoms. Sometimes an individual may simply be given the diagnosis of a form of incontinence, so we've covered the different types of urinary incontinence also (Chapter 5).

Chapter 8 describes the kinds of medical investigations that you might undergo in order to gain a diagnosis. You may have already experienced some of these and find the information familiar. If you're on the start of your journey with bladder problems and have an investigation coming up, you may want to read this chapter first. There are signposts to other chapters which you can go back to later.

Chapters 9 to 11 discuss behavioural treatments, such as pelvic floor exercises, what food and drinks frequently trigger bladder symptoms and changes you can make in daily life to ease bladder discomfort. Next, in Chapters 12 and 13, we look at medications and surgical procedures for urinary problems. Because the symptoms of bladder conditions often overlap, we haven't divided the chapters on treatment in terms of each diagnosis; rather, we've grouped different types of treatments and therapies together. We would recommend that you try the dietary, exercise and lifestyle advice first to see if symptoms reduce or resolve from these changes. All medications and surgical procedures pose side effects and risks so, if possible, it's best to use these types of interventions only if the things you can do yourself don't help to get symptoms under control.

In Chapter 14, we've reviewed the scientific evidence for complementary and alternative medicine (CAM) in bladder health. You may also want to consider these therapies in addition to your medical treatments, before embarking on an invasive procedure, or if you feel you've tried the orthodox options already. We strongly advise you tell your GP or specialist when/ if you start a CAM therapy so that they have a complete picture of your health activities.

Finally, we end the book with a chapter on additional things you can do to support your bladder and overall health. These include practical tips on how to access toilets when out, discreet products and general advice on how to manage stress and get a good night's sleep.

We sincerely hope you find this book useful.

Chapter 1

You are not alone: bladder problems are very common

Respondents reported stigma associated with urinary frequency and urgency, not just UI [urinary infection]. In particular, they reported feelings of embarrassment and shame associated with having to make frequent trips to the bathroom when in the company of others.

Elstad and colleagues (2010)[18]

In this chapter we discuss:
- how common bladder problems are and how they affect people's lives
- the reasons why this type of health issue is still stigmatised in Western society
- how the bladder and bowel work and how these organs affect, and interact with, one another (People often have problems with both the bladder and the bowel so knowing how these organs are interconnected can help understanding of this symptom.)
- the impact of sleep disruption due to bladder problems, and
- how lack of understanding and support from family and friends can affect life for people with both bladder and bowel issues.

How common are bladder problems ('bladder dysfunction')?

Approximately 14 million people in the UK live with some form of bladder complaint. This equates to over 20% of the population, so even if you don't personally experience the embarrassing and intrusive symptoms of bladder dysfunction, it is likely that you know someone who does.

Bladder problems are common throughout the world. In 2010, a study found that in Sweden, overactive bladder syndrome (OAB) created problems for around 15% of men, and 34% of women.[1] The percentages for the UK were slightly less at 11% of men and 23% of women, but this is still more than one in 10 men and nearly a quarter of women in the UK.

One study, several years ago,[2] reported the prevalence of OAB in a random sample of the population in six European countries. This included the percentage of men and women over the age of 40 who had the symptoms of OAB. The figures were as follows:

France	12%	(estimated to affect 2.9 million)
Germany	18%	6.5 million
Italy	12%	3.3 million
Spain	22%	3.6 million
Sweden	19%	0.8 million
UK	20%	5.2 million

Apart from these countries, the sheer number of studies on bladder dysfunction by teams in countries all over the globe shows that this problem affects millions worldwide – for example, in 2005 the prevalence in Japan for OAB was 14% of men and 11% of women.[3] A recent study in Turkey estimated that the prevalence of OAB in women was 21%.[4]

People who do not have bladder dysfunction

Most people who haven't (yet) had bladder problems don't even think about their bladder. If everything is working correctly, the bladder gradually fills up until the person feels the need to urinate (pee). Generally, the bladder can hold between 300 and 600 millilitres (ml) of urine, but the urge to go to the toilet is triggered before the bladder is full. People differ in the size of their bladder, how much it can hold, and how long they can wait until they are not able to hold on. The average healthy person with no bladder problems will probably need to pee between four and seven times a day, and generally not need to get up during the night to 'go'.

Many people associate bladder problems with getting older, but unfortunately the bladder does not discriminate as these problems affect all ages, including children. However, on average, men and women show differences in the way they deal with problems. Nancy Muller, researching in the USA, found that 71% of men and 61% of women had never discussed their bladder health with a doctor.[5] In Western societies, men do seem more reluctant to see a doctor, not only for bladder problems but for other health issues too.

> *Men are less aware of their symptoms than women, and are more reluctant to seek help.*
>
> Peter Baker, Chief Executive
> of the Men's Health Forum, BBC News[6]

Considering age as a potential factor, although older people are more likely to suffer from such problems, it is not a natural part of ageing. Nancy Muller found that the majority of people in her sample believed that loss of bladder control first occurs in people aged around 60. However, the truth is that those who have symptoms actually start experiencing them in their 40s. On the other hand, older women are more likely to consult their doctors than women in their 20s and 30s.

Despite the fact that these health issues are very common, it can be difficult to discuss them with your family, friends and even your doctor. Many people suffer needlessly in silence even though there is now a wide range of investigations that can lead to effective and long-lasting symptom relief. This book will guide you through the different conditions associated with bladder dysfunction, what to expect if you need to undergo investigations and the numerous treatments that are available so that you will no longer need to feel reluctant to broach the subject with your GP – meaning you can find your way back to good health.

Why do some people have problems with their bladder?

There are many reasons why people have problems with their bladder, but there often seems to be no reason why someone develops bladder symptoms. However, the symptoms of many bladder disorders are associated with anxiety and depression, including:

- a sudden urge to pee, especially if there is no toilet nearby
- worry about possible urine leakage
- having to go to pee multiple times during the day, with the associated worry that people will notice
- having to get up in the night to pee, causing sleep loss
- feeling that the symptoms are embarrassing and worrying
- social and other relationships being affected.

I remember that I used to go out dancing and I would try not to drink too much and then I would go to the loo all the time to empty my bladder before the dance but it wouldn't make any difference. It used to be embarrassing because, you know, anything I wore got wet; then it was embarrassing going in someone's car afterwards so it really ruled my life.

Denny

An additional problem is that people with bladder problems are more likely to have bowel problems as well. This works both ways – for example, people with irritable bowel syndrome (IBS) are more likely than others to have bladder problems.[7]

The bladder and the bowel are related; Figure 1 shows how close the bowel and the bladder are to each other.

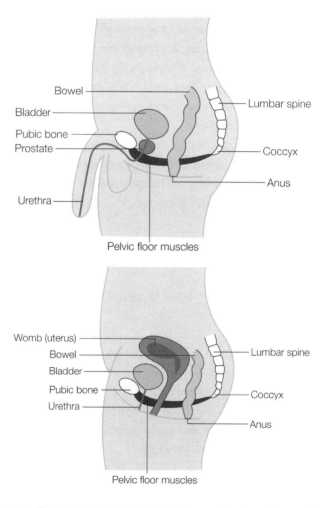

Figure 1: The position of the urinary system and the bowel in men (top) and women, showing how close they are

Distension of the bowel affects the bladder, and vice versa. As we have said, people with bladder problems often find that they also have bowel dysfunction. Peter Whorwell and colleagues, back in 1986, studying people with IBS, noted that many of their patients also had bladder problems.[8]

This has been confirmed in many other studies. In 2015, researchers in Norway confirmed that the bladder could affect, and be affected by, the bowel.[9] People with IBS often complain that their bladder is sensitive, and people with bladder problems complain of constipation. People who have both problems should first try to sort out the constipation problem (see Chapter 11, page 128-130). Relieving constipation often helps with the overactive bladder problem.

When patients have radiation therapy for bladder cancer, bowel problems are common. Urgency to poo, diarrhoea and poo leakage are of course extremely distressing symptoms, which have a large impact on a person's quality of life.

Why is it that bladder problems are hard to talk about?

Bladder dysfunction can lead to people having anxieties in their social lives and relationships. The symptoms can also be embarrassing. This is rather like IBS. Often people with IBS cannot simply go out and enjoy themselves without first knowing where toilets are located. In respect of the bladder, Nancy Muller found that 62% of her sample said they routinely looked out for toilets when they were, for instance, visiting an amusement park. People with the problem also make sure they know the location of toilets when they go out generally.

Bladder problems have plagued me now for 50+ years. I still find it embarrassing to have to go to the toilet so often. When I am out, I need to locate the nearest toilet, I book seats on planes next to toilets. Whilst working as a teacher, I found it very hard to be tied to a classroom knowing I could not leave it to go to the toilet when I needed to, as I could not leave the children on their own. As my bladder problems have gone on so long, I have become more stressed over time about needing to go to the toilet but one not being promptly available. My bladder habits are something of a family joke, but that does nothing to reduce the stress I feel!

Sharon

Some people feel insecure in public toilets, and wait until they are alone before using one. They are worried about the smell of urine, that others might realise they have bladder problems, and that they might leak urine.

I hear a lot of women talking about how 'I just don't want to be a smelly old woman' as soon as they are pregnant. But in the last trimester, when they're heavily pregnant, most women would leak a bit when they're laughing or on the trampoline and it's a thing that's of such concern that they automatically start fretting about, you know, having odour issues when they're older. But this doesn't have to be the case as physio is so effective.

Elaine Miller, physiotherapist and comedian

Having to carry a change of clothes, or wearing pads, was also a worry. Needless to say, this is an additional stress. Many, many people have bladder problems but have never consulted a doctor; they have no diagnosis, and therefore no treatments to help them. Those who have a diagnosis, however, are likely to manage better. Having said that, in the USA, Nancy Muller found that on average women experienced symptoms for 6.5 years before being diagnosed, while men waited 4.2 years.

In our other self-help books (see page vii), we have shown how irritable bowel syndrome (IBS), CFS/ME and other chronic illnesses can lead to people feeling stigmatised. Studies have shown that people with bowel or bladder problems feel embarrassment and shame, which means they are less likely to want to admit to having such problems – even to their GP.

A question of dignity

I've been looking into incontinence in different societies and there seems to be something visceral about not having control of your body. It seems to be associated with people who are very, very young, very, very ill or incompetent in some way. It's human dignity, isn't it?

Elaine Miller

The word 'incontinence', by its very definition, means loss of control which is something that taps into our sense of dignity. But is soiling yourself worse than dying? This may seem like a trite question, but in a notable study which asked 180 people who were over 60 years old and with a serious illness that required hospitalisation about this, it seemed that the fear of incontinence was worse than the fear of death.[10] These patients were asked whether a number of debilitating circumstances would be worse than dying. These circumstances included being in constant moderate pain, being confined to a wheelchair, relying on a feeding tube, being confused all the time and being bladder and bowel incontinent. For almost 70% of those questioned, not being able to control their bladder and bowel was seen as a fate worse than death. This tells us a bit about how deeply we feel about losing control of our bodies, in particular being able to control going to the toilet; this seems to be a question of dignity, which is a fundamental part of human experience.

Bladder cancer

Researchers Heyes and colleagues, in relation to people with bladder cancer, examined six articles where study participants had undergone 'intravesical therapy' (the instillation of chemotherapy or immunotherapy agents into the bladder) or the surgical formation of a stoma or 'neobladder'.[11] The researchers looked at the themes that were important to people with bladder cancer. These were:

- communication and information
- sexuality
- shock and fear of diagnosis
- treatment and recovery
- life after surgery
- body image
- support and comfort.

Although this study was about bladder cancer, the themes of communication and information, and, body image and sexuality, are of course important for people who have less serious bladder conditions.

Communication and information

It's important that doctors take you seriously. In Heyes and colleagues' study, some people believed that clinicians doubted them, or minimised their symptoms. Some doctors used terms which were confusing, and sometimes different doctors were giving patients different information about treatment. People also wanted to hear from other people with the same problem. Support from doctors, family and friends was very important. Indeed, people who had a supportive doctor and where both the patient and doctor treated bladder conditions as a long-term illness, fared better.[12]

Body image

As we have seen from the stories in this chapter, and those in our other books, having a chronic illness – especially one which involves bowel or bladder symptoms – takes a toll on body image. People find it difficult to trust their bodies, they have to get used to being a person who is unwell, and maybe who cannot do things which they did before. They grieve for the person they used to be. Urgency to get to the toilet, fearing leakage, having incontinence – this can undermine their sense of self. This is especially true for people with bladder cancer. A study in China showed that the prevalence of depressive and anxiety symptoms was 78% in patients with this condition.[13] It's common to feel anxious and depressed with bladder problems, especially so for bladder cancer. We talk more about how to cope with this anxiety in Chapter 15.

Sexuality

Society expects that people should be able to control their bodily functions, and also have a sense of sexuality. However, often people with bladder cancer, especially if they have a stoma, feel that they are sexually unappealing, are embarrassed, and find social and sexual relationships are not easy. Participants in the study above by Heyes and colleagues[11] said that they had lost self-respect and confidence. It is important to note, however, that some couples had overcome these difficulties, although it had taken some time. This is almost bound to be the case, as people have to adapt to new roles, whilst grieving for their life pre-surgery.

It is not only people with bladder cancer who find sexuality difficult. Bladder dysfunction may also lead to sexual problems. This might be because sexual activity can cause an urgent need to pee, and also to urinary leakage. Fears of this happening can lead to avoiding sexual activity, which may also contribute to feeling bad. People with overactive bladder (OAB – see Chapter 5, page 51) and interstitial cystitis (IC – see Chapter 6, page 64) often find sex painful. Sexual activity can also trigger bladder contractions. One study found that between 49% and 90% of women questioned found it painful.[14] Half of adults who were sexually active said that their OAB symptoms affected their relationship with their partner, and that their enjoyment of sex was reduced.[15] Another study found that 54% of women with chronic bladder disorders avoided intimacy with their partners most of the time.[16] Unfortunately, many women find it difficult to broach this subject with health professionals, and many health professionals don't find it easy to address these issues. Thus, women who would like help often don't receive it. The lack of intimacy can lead of feelings of alienation and depression.

Researchers in Vienna investigated the impact of OAB on sexual relationships in both men and women. The study included a total of around 1000 men and 1000 women, ranging from 19 to 91 years. The overall prevalence of OAB was 14%.[17] The researchers found that nearly 18% of people with OAB reported a negative impact on their sexual life. OAB is often sub-typed into 'OAB-wet' (this group have urgency incontinence) or 'OAB-dry' (this group do not have urgency incontinence). The people with OAB-wet reported more of an impact on sexual life than the OAB-dry group.

Quality of life

On average, people who have to live with a chronic illness do not have such a good quality of life as people who are healthy. Bladder problems (often with concurrent bowel symptoms) are difficult to deal with, and people who have to cope with these are usually well aware that their quality of life has been diminished.

One factor which causes quality of life to be reduced is the stigma and taboo which are attached to certain illnesses. These are the negative emotions people feel when they have something about them that they perceive to be shameful or unacceptable. Some illnesses are more acceptable than others, and therefore they differ in the extent to which people with such illnesses feel stigmatised. For instance, cancer is less stigmatised than AIDS. Stigma is also associated with depression and anxiety – on average, the more the person feels stigmatised, the more depression and anxiety they feel. So we can begin to see why people with bladder problems might feel anxious and depressed.

Studies show that when people have problems that relate to toilet habits, such as IBS or inflammatory bowel disease (IBD), they feel higher levels of stigmatisation. This leads to their quality of life being worse than people who do not feel stigmatised.

In 2010, researchers Emily Elstad and colleagues carried out a study which showed that higher frequency and urgency to pee were a source of stigma, which was linked to anxiety, depression and hopelessness.[18] They said that frequency and urgency affected people on a social, not just physical, level. This was because they often had to make frequent trips to the toilet in the presence of others, which drew attention to them and their private body parts.

There are different types of bladder problems, which we discuss in Chapters 5–7. The most common complaint, an overactive bladder (OAB), is accompanied by urinary urgency or incontinence (leaking of urine). Studies have shown, perhaps unsurprisingly, that urinary incontinence is the most distressing aspect of having a problematic bladder. This can lead to depression and a reduced quality of life.

People with chronic illness often try to hide their symptoms from others, because they feel ashamed, think others will laugh or stigmatise them, or blame them because they think they should be able to control themselves:

I don't hide my symptoms from others because it is very clear that I am always rushing off to the loo. If I could hide my problems, life would be far less embarrassing. Many people are negative about my bladder problems, expecting me to be able to control them, when I can't.

Sharon

I did hide it all and felt very, very ashamed. Maybe if I'd had a baby then people would have been okay because everyone knows that childbirth can affect your bladder and bowels. I hid my symptoms from everyone for a long time – until I had the op that actually showed something. I don't think people believed me. I did feel ashamed and embarrassed – what's worse, that or not being in control of your bladder? (Apart from your bowel!)

Sarah

One study in 1993 found that 70% of people with painful bladder syndrome said that their family relationships and responsibilities had been affected, and that employment was difficult or impossible in 84%.[19]

Many people suffer in silence because they feel embarrassed to talk to their GP, believe that there is no treatment or think it's just that they are getting old. However, there are treatments which can help. So, we would encourage anyone who feels embarrassed to be brave and go to their GP.

Pain

All bladder problems are likely to have associated pain. Depending on the type of bladder complaint, the pain can be variable – that is, mild to severe, occurring most of the time or intermittently. It is therefore really helpful to have supportive people who understand your complaint, and who can help you through the bad times (see social support, page 176). Women with bladder pain (interstitial cystitis – IC) have urinary frequency and urgency. This condition has been shown to lead to a decrease in mental and physical health.

Sleep

Many people without bladder problems sometimes have to get up in the night to pee. However, people with bladder problems often have to get up *multiple* times in the night, which disturbs sleep; incontinence may also be a problem, and these together can become a very distressing symptom. One study looked at the sleep of 3397 people with both general bladder problems and IC (also called 'painful bladder syndrome'). It found that half of the sample of people interviewed reported bad sleep quality, and 615 reported that they had less than six hours' sleep per night.[20] Participants reported that sleep was affected due to having to get up to pee in the night, or trouble sleeping due to bladder pain.

Altogether, 50% of the sample reported 'fairly bad' or 'very bad' sleep quality, and 61% reported sleep duration of less than six hours. In people with IC, the most prevalent symptom was trouble sleeping 'due to the need to use the bathroom' (59%), with 44% of the sample reporting trouble sleeping due to urgency, and 22% due to bladder pain.

> I have slept poorly for years, as I need to use the toilet several times in the night. This in turn makes me constantly tired.
>
> *Sharon*

The medical name for getting up in the night to 'void' (empty your bladder) is 'nocturia'. This can be part of many bladder conditions. Research looking into overactive bladder syndrome (OAB; Chapter 5, page 51) found that women who had nocturia were fatigued in the day, and had a decreased quality of life and sleep, with associated low mood.[21] These problems were increased, the more often the woman had to get up in the night. The study also found that nocturia led to increased sick leave and lower productivity.

Poor sleep is associated with worse physical health, depression and a decreased quality of life. Whilst there is medication to help with sleep, there are other ways of trying to improve sleep quality, which might be worth trying first (see Chapter 15, page 178).

Social support

Having a bladder condition can affect all aspects of life. It is therefore helpful to have people around you who understand your problems. We have shown in our other books how important social support is, especially for people with chronic illness. The support of other people isn't just a psychological boost for us. The effect is partially hormonal. As we say in our book on IBS:

> *Oxytocin is a hormone which is secreted by the pituitary gland in the brain... oxytocin is released when you feel supported by others. Studies have shown that oxytocin and social support interact together in reducing cortisol (a stress hormone) which means that stress is reduced.*
>
> Arroll and Dancey[22]

Researchers in Canada found that having the support of a partner decreased the negative impact of pain on the mental quality of life in women with bladder dysfunction.[23]

Not everyone will experience high levels of social support, though. Regarding Sharon's family, she says:

I would like them [my family] to know that my bladder problems have plagued me for most of my life. They are real and interfere greatly with day-to-day activities. When they treat them as a joke, they fail to realise how painful and uncomfortable the symptoms are. This makes me feel even more like I should be able to control the symptoms, despite most avenues of treatment having failed me.

Sharon

Summary and conclusion

In this first chapter, we have touched on what it's like to have a bladder condition – the difficulties people can face and why incontinence can be so very hard to talk about. Bladder conditions can affect our body image, sexuality and overall quality of life, yet these things can be extremely hard to speak about. We hope that this book not only explains some of the reasons why bladder problems develop, but also allows you to find the help (both medical and support from family and friends) that you deserve. In Chapter 2, we outline the anatomy of the urinary system because having some awareness of this can make it easier to understand why our bladders may stop working properly.

Chapter 2

The bladder – what is it and what does it do?

Like all the organs in our body, we really don't notice the bladder until something starts to go wrong with it, or we begin to experience symptoms. Furthermore, we can often go for a very long time with unpleasant symptoms before we seek help from a doctor; of course, many symptoms do resolve on their own.

To help us understand the problems that occur in this organ, this chapter explores the structure and function of the bladder and kidneys which together make up the urinary system. We hope that this will make it much easier to understand the conditions that can develop, as described later in the book.

The bladder

The bladder can be thought of as a storage sack for urine – but that is a rather simplistic representation. Like all of the structures in our bodies, it is a complex organ that communicates with our brain in order to keep functioning. When It is working properly it doesn't bother us until it is nearing its capacity. Otherwise we would feel the need to wee constantly! But this does happen with conditions such as interstitial cystitis (IC; Chapter 6, page 64) where inflammation in the bladder triggers signals to the brain that the bladder needs to be emptied even when there isn't much urine to pass. People with IC know how difficult life can be when they feel they need to be near a toilet constantly. Luckily for people without any bladder issues, it's taken for granted that their brains will tell them when they need to urinate.

Before the age of 10 I led a normal life. I was a typical child, went to school every day, had fun going around and about with my friends. I enjoyed going on school trips and always loved to see different places, I loved swimming just simply to immerse myself in crystal blue sea and feel the bliss. Nothing was a problem to me; I loved outdoors, I loved going to Mass even if it lasted a very long time. I had freedom.

All of this changed one morning. I got up, dressed for school, ate breakfast, drank my favourite hot drink (which is I believe the favourite drink of most 10-year-old children), a cocoa. I went to the school feeling very happy as it was my last day of lessons before the winter/Christmas holidays. Out of the blue, my life changed forever – though I did not know then what I know now. I had never had bladder problems before so I was scared when that day I had to go all the time; I went, came back, and got the urge again; I had to go to the ladies' room so fast as I thought I would not make it, the urge was so big. I felt irritation in the bladder. I was very frightened and worried and ashamed. I did not know what to think.

Martina

As Martina mentions in her narrative, before she started to have bladder problems she really wasn't aware of her urinary system at all.

The urinary system

The bladder is part of the renal (or urinary) system, which also includes the kidneys, ureters and the urethra (see Figure 2). The entire function of this bodily system is to produce, store and finally eliminate our fluid waste product (urine), but like all the systems in our bodies, it doesn't work in isolation. The renal system interacts with the lungs, intestines and even our skin in order to keep an optimal balance of water and other substances (such as sodium, phosphorus and potassium) in our bodies.

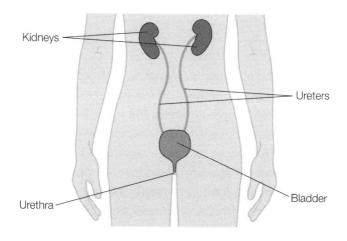

Figure 2: The urinary system

The kidneys

The renal system begins with the kidneys, which filter potentially harmful substances from our blood. Their work allows the body to maintain homeostasis (a balanced state, or equilibrium), which is vital for our health. Our bodies must maintain equilibrium in terms of essential mechanisms such as blood pressure, glucose levels in our blood and core temperature, otherwise we cannot function – in fact we would eventually die if any of these mechanisms was disturbed for an extended period of time. But when all of our physiological systems are stable we are said to be in a state of homeostasis. The kidneys play an essential part in maintaining this balance. They achieve this by acting as active filters using the many thousands of functional units called nephrons (see below) of which they are made up. (The study of the kidneys is known as nephrology.)

However, many things can go wrong with our kidneys and people who have damaged kidneys may have to use a dialysis machine, otherwise waste products that can't be eliminated will build up in their bodies and become toxic.

Nephrons

There are around a million nephrons in each kidney but as we get older this number declines. These tiny structures are very important as they eliminate waste from our bodies. They do this via two structures, called the glomerulus and the kidney (or 'renal') tubule (see Figure 3). The glomerulus is the actual blood 'filter' and is formed of a tiny blood vessel – capillary – which is wound up around itself very tightly, like a bit like a ball of wool. We can think of this structure as a sieve that leaves normal proteins, electrolytes, macronutrients and some water in the bloodstream but takes out excess electrolytes, micronutrients, toxins and waste products. The glomerulus passes these waste products on to the tubule (tiny tube). Here the wastes are filtered out and passed to the bladder via the ureters, the two narrow tubes that link the kidneys with the bladder. The kidneys actively measure concentrations of substances like sodium, phosphorus and potassium and release the amounts we require back into the bloodstream if and when we need them, to preserve homeostasis. Therefore, the kidneys control the levels of electrolytes and water in the body, passing out what is not needed as urine.

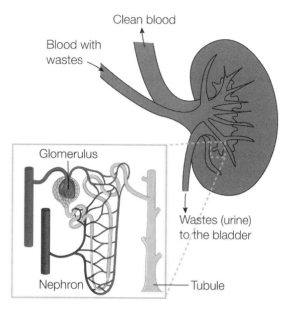

Figure 3: The components of the kidney

Common kidney problems

Conditions involving the kidneys have risen in recent years, possibly due to the increase in chronic conditions such as obesity and diabetes that can affect these organs.[24] The most frequent problems with the kidneys include:

- Kidney disease – This is really an umbrella term for any kidney abnormality, most cases of which will be relatively mild. However, some people can develop what's known as 'kidney failure' and if this is the case, dialysis treatment or a kidney transplant may be required. The term 'chronic kidney disease' or 'CKD' is often used as this group of conditions are 'managed', rather than 'cured', and are often 'progressive' (worsen over time).

- Kidney infections – These occur where bacteria that have made their way to the bladder continue on into the kidneys. Symptoms can include: pain when going to the toilet (weeing), blood in the urine, urine appearing cloudy and/or having a strong smell, and sometimes having a fever. These symptoms are very much like those of a bladder infection, so do see your doctor who will be able to diagnose what the problem is and give appropriate treatment (usually a course of antibiotics to kill off the bacteria).

- Kidney stones (nephrolithiasis) – These are like small pebbles or crystals that have built up in the kidneys. They are made of substances such as calcium and uric acid and can be as tiny as a grain of salt or as large as a golf ball. The small ones often simply pass when you wee, but bigger ones can cause a significant amount of pain and may need to be removed by surgery (often keyhole surgery). Although in themselves the stones aren't problematic, if they get stuck in the kidney or ureter (see below) your doctor will most likely want to remove them. Symptoms of kidney stones include pain (can be severe) around the back or at the side of the stomach, which can radiate to the groin area.
- Kidney cancer – Like kidney disease, kidney cancer is also on the rise. In the past decade, there has been an increase of around a third and it is the eighth most common type of cancer in the UK and USA.
- Acute kidney injury (AKI) – This is not caused by a kick to the side of the body as is inferred by the name; rather, it is usually the result of another serious condition, such as heart or liver failure and so is mostly seen only in older people. This acute condition differs from chronic kidney disease as people can recover fully from it, as opposed to the chronic nature of CKD.

The ureters

Once the nephrons have done their job and filtered our blood of potentially damaging substances, the resulting urine then passes down the renal tubules of each kidney towards the ureters. These thin structures are between 20 and 25 centimetres (8-10 inches) long. They are continuously contracting and relaxing, a motion that forces the urine towards the bladder and away from the kidneys. All this perpetual motion goes on in our bodies throughout the day and night – it's amazing really when you think of how hard our bodies work for us without our knowledge. We only really become aware of these things of course when they stop working properly, but if all is well, then the ureters expel small volumes of urine into the bladder every 10 to 15 seconds.

The bladder

So now we come to the bladder itself. The bladder is positioned in the pelvic cavity, in front of the rectum and behind the reproductive organs of the pelvis. If you think about it for a moment, the bladder is very much nestled between other important structures of the body, and in women it shares a restricted area in the pelvic cavity with the uterus (womb). In fact, the uterus rests above and next to the bladder, which is why pregnant women often feel the need to use the toilet more often when the expanding uterus squeezes the available space. Women also tend to have smaller bladders than men and so cannot hold the same volume of urine, but the amount of fluid we can each individually hold does vary. However, on average the bladder can accommodate anywhere between 300 and 600 millilitres of liquid due to its elastic qualities. Importantly, a healthy, properly functioning bladder can hold this volume of urine for a number of hours – up to five – without any problems.

The bladder is able to expand to hold these amounts of fluid because it is made up of three layers of separate types of tissue – the mucosa, submucosa and the muscularis layer (also called the 'detrusor muscle', see Figure 4, page 33) – that have the ability to expand and contract, thereby holding urine for relatively long periods of time. People often simply refer to the detrusor muscle when talking about the bladder and urination, as this is the layer that contracts and relaxes when going to the toilet.

The sphincters

Importantly, the passing of urine through the bladder is controlled by circular muscles called sphincters (internal and external). The 'internal urethral sphincter' is a circle of muscle that surrounds the urethral opening (the opening at the bottom of the bladder) and holds urine in. This mechanism, unlike the external sphincter, is not under our conscious control but rather the brain directs its action automatically. However, the external (or 'distal') urethral sphincter is controlled voluntarily by us, via the somatic nervous system (see page 27). So in effect, there are two ways – conscious/voluntary and unconscious/automatic – in which our bodies prevent urinary incontinence.

If the sphincter function is compromised – for instance, if communication between the brain and bladder becomes impaired (see Chapter 3) – then urine may leak out, resulting in incontinence.

The urethra

The urethra is the tube that runs from the bladder to the outside of the body. It is positioned at the bottom of the bladder and in women the external opening lies between the clitoris and vagina while in men it is at the end of the penis.

Not only do women tend to have smaller bladders than men, but their urethras are also normally much shorter (3.8-5.1 cm/1.5-2 inches compared with 20 cm/8 inches). A short urethra can be a problem as bacteria can enter more easily and pass back into the bladder, causing a urinary tract infection (UTI) or cystitis (see Chapter 6). In other words, there is a considerable difference in the distance between the bladder and bacteria on the skin in men and women, hence the more common occurrence of cystitis in women than men.

The pelvic floor muscles

The pelvic floor muscles can be thought of as a hammock which supports not only the bladder but also the bowels and, in women, the uterus (see Figure 1, page 5). As well as keeping the urethra closed until you're ready to go to the toilet, the pelvic floor muscles also stop urine leaking when you cough or sneeze and control the discharge of wind.

The pelvic floor muscles can become weakened or damaged during the course of life. Childbirth, obesity, strenuous exercise and lifting heavy objects, or even the repeated straining that happens when someone has chronic constipation, can affect this group of muscles. These muscles also slacken with age. As you can see from Figure 1, the pelvic floor muscles stretch from our tailbone (coccyx), which is just above our bottom, to the pubic bone at the front of our bodies. Healthy pelvic floor muscles are thick and quite firm and, like any muscle, their tone can be improved – which is very good news as this is something we can tackle ourselves with targeted exercises (see Chapter 9, page 102).

How many times a day should I empty my bladder?

The ideal number of times to empty the bladder in a day of course differs between people, and bladder sizes vary somewhat, but on average a healthy person may urinate between four and eight times a day. Perhaps more important than the number of times we visit the toilet are the colour and smell of our urine as these can tell us if we're drinking enough fluid. If our wee is very dark and has a strong smell we are probably dehydrated. Proper hydration is important for overall health so, if this is the case, consider increasing your fluid intake, but avoid caffeinated drinks as these have diuretic qualities which encourage the kidneys to pull water from our bodies to be passed via the bladder. While this is not a damaging process, and indeed diuretic products are often suggested for people with high blood pressure and cardiovascular conditions, if you're dehydrated this can lead to fatigue, sleepiness and headaches and put you in a bad mood.

On the other hand, being overhydrated doesn't usually have anything to do with drinking too much fluid as the kidneys will simply kick-in and excrete anything that the body doesn't need. If your urine is very pale or even looks exactly like water you may want to reduce the amount you drink to maintain the correct balance of salts and minerals in the body, which we need to function. Pale-straw-coloured urine is a sign of good, but not over, hydration.

Summary and conclusion

In this chapter, we have presented a great deal of information, starting with a description of the bladder and renal system before moving on to some behavioural advice about how often we should go to the toilet. It's all quite technical but we have explored the anatomy and physiology of the urinary system here because we believe it's important to understand the structure and function of an organ that's causing problems so that we can then appreciate how treatments work. We hope that this sets the scene for understanding bladder issues, so that effective and sustainable relief may be found.

In the next chapter, we describe how we know when to go to the toilet – that is, how the bladder and brain communicate.

Chapter 3

How does the bladder communicate with the brain?

In Chapter 2 we looked at the structure of the bladder and its function within the renal system. Of course, the bladder doesn't work on its own – our brain must tell us when we need to go to the toilet, via signals from the bladder. This is important as sometimes this signalling goes awry (see Chapter 5) and so rather than treating the bladder directly, the correct course of action could be to remedy this pathway. Therefore, in this chapter, we look at how the bladder and brain communicate with each other, and with the urinary system as a whole. To start, we briefly outline key areas of the nervous system that play a part in this.

Central and peripheral nervous systems

The central nervous system, or CNS, comprises the brain and spinal cord. In addition, we have a system that allows our organs to communicate with our brain, known as the peripheral nervous system.[25] This system can be separated into three parts: the somatic, autonomic and enteric nervous systems.

Somatic nervous system

The somatic nervous system controls voluntary actions (that is, body movements within our conscious awareness) and consists of all the neurons (nerve cells) connected with skeletal muscles and skin. In addition, the somatic nervous system is the gateway between the outside world and our experience of it. Receptors for external stimuli inform the CNS of what's going on around us via our senses of sight, smell, taste, hearing and touch. In addition, the somatic nervous system gives sensory information to the CNS about the goings-on of our internal organs (our internal world). This includes the awareness of how full our bladder is.

Autonomic nervous system

Unlike the somatic nervous system, the autonomic nervous system controls involuntary processes that are outside our conscious awareness. The name for this system refers to this – that is, it works autonomously, so it doesn't take any conscious effort from us and thereby appears 'automatic'. The bodily functions influenced by the autonomic nervous system include the heart rate, pupil dilation, perspiration and respiration. This system is further sub-divided into the **sympathetic** and **parasympathetic** nervous systems.

Sympathetic nervous system

The sympathetic nervous system controls how we respond to a threat, known as the 'fight or flight' response. This is also called the 'stress response' as our bodies respond to a threat or stressor when needed by readying our muscles, hearts and lungs to flee or contend with whatever is threatening our safety. In our ancestors' times, this would have been a dangerous animal or rival clan but now it's more likely to be an event or a difficult situation. For example, many people feel the need to wee frequently just before something like giving a public speech. This is because the sympathetic nervous system is doing its best to make escape or defending oneself as successful as possible; one aspect of this is to eliminate waste as soon as possible so that you don't have to stop for a toilet break halfway through the encounter.

Parasympathetic nervous system

The parasympathetic nervous system is the opposite side of the same coin in terms of the autonomic (unconscious) nervous system. It restores the body back to a state of equilibrium, or 'homeostasis'. As opposed to the fight-or-flight response, the parasympathetic nervous system is involved in the 'rest and digest' response once a stressful situation has passed. Here, the heart rate will slow back down, our muscles will relax again and we are able to rest.

Enteric nervous system

The enteric nervous system relates to the nerves of the gut. Although the enteric nervous system is not involved directly in urination ('micturition', see below), we mention it here as the next chapter explores the subject of the gut microbiota (the microbe system in our large bowel) and the 'brain-gut axis'. These have been shown in many research studies to be important with regard to a vast range of illnesses and chronic conditions, including bladder problems.

Working together

To summarise up to this point, the central nervous system communicates with our bodies via the sensory and autonomic nervous systems that are part of the peripheral nervous system. The important 'take home' message here is that in order to go to the toilet, we need both voluntary and involuntary (conscious and unconscious – sensory and autonomic) messages to control the external urethral sphincter.

In the next section, we outline the actual process that allows us to urinate; this is called 'urination/micturition'.

Micturition

Micturition, the medical term for urination, is made up of a complex set of mechanisms that involve the nervous systems mentioned above. Several reflexes are also fundamental to this mechanism; these are either inhibited (red traffic light) or facilitated (green traffic light) by our brain.[26] There are two key stages in this process:

Stage 1: The storage phase – The bladder fills gradually – small amounts of urine are dripped into the bladder throughout the day, but this in itself doesn't prompt us to use the toilet. During this time, tension in the bladder walls progressively increases with the addition of more and more urine and the bladder will be relaxed – that is, you will not feel the need to go to the toilet.

Stage 2: The voiding phase – The following nervous reflexes are triggered:

   a. the micturition reflex that gives us the conscious desire to urinate;

   b. the autonomic spinal cord reflex – this is either inhibited or facilitated by the brain to allow us to 'hold it' or empty the bladder;

   c. the detrusor muscle contracts, opening the external sphincter so that urine can be excreted via the urethra (though we can override this consciously).

Micturition reflex

In the previous chapter we described the bladder as a storage vessel, a bit like an empty sack or balloon that can fill up. But how do we know when it's reaching its limit in terms of urine volume (known as the 'threshold volume') and needs to be emptied?

The bladder wall houses sensory nerve receptors that detect tension, or stretch. This is why the somatic nervous system is important in micturition. When the bladder is at about half of its capacity (around 200-300 ml of urine) these receptors are activated and send signals along the pelvic nerve to the spinal cord and brain. Then a reflex signal is pinged back to the bladder, specifically the detrusor muscle, which causes the bladder wall to contract. When the bladder wall contracts there is an increased sensation of pressure and that sensation is what makes us want to wee. When there isn't too much urine in the bladder, in other words when the bladder volume is low, this communication between the brain and the bladder tells us that we'll be okay to wait awhile before we find a toilet. However, when the bladder becomes fuller the urge to wee gets stronger and it can become very uncomfortable until urination occurs, offering relief.

On average, the micturition reflex occurs four to eight times a day, depending on how much a person drinks. Importantly for people with bladder issues, the micturition reflex can be triggered by either an involuntary or a voluntary action.

Involuntary action

If the threshold volume of the bladder is reached and exceeded, the peripheral nervous system can trigger the micturition reflex outside our conscious control – that is, we can have an accident and urinate without wanting too. This could simply be because we were trying to avoid going to the loo, for instance if we are not near a toilet, or there can be problems with the nerves and sensory fibres in the bladder wall (see pages 33–34), leading to incontinence.

Voluntary action

However, people without bladder problems usually urinate voluntarily, under their conscious control. Here, the CNS and brain can tell the muscles we describe next to empty the bladder even when it has not reached the volume threshold and there isn't much urine to pass. Often people go to the loo before a trip so that their bladder has more space to fill over the journey time, hence in most circumstances we can go to the toilet when we choose.

Muscles involved in micturition

We looked at the structure and function of the bladder in Chapter 2 and introduced the detrusor muscle, the internal and external urethral sphincters and the pelvic floor muscles. All of these muscles play an important part in micturition and are controlled by the autonomic and somatic nervous systems. For someone to urinate, the following muscular actions take place:

- the internal sphincter is tense when the bladder is filling during the storage phase, while the detrusor muscle is relaxed, thereby retaining the bladder's contents;
- when the bladder reaches its threshold volume the detrusor muscle contracts;
- in the voiding phase of micturition, the internal sphincter starts to relax;
- then the external sphincter also relaxes either under conscious, voluntary control or unconscious, involuntary control (above); and
- the pelvic floor relaxes too so that the urethra can open, allowing urine to be passed (see Figure 4).

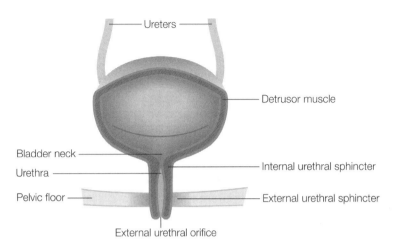

Ureters

Detrusor muscle

Bladder neck

Internal urethral sphincter

Urethra

Pelvic floor

External urethral sphincter

External urethral orifice

Figure 4: The muscles that control micturition (urination)

Problems that can occur in brain–bladder communication

Like any form of two-way communication, the messages between the brain and bladder can be disrupted. This can be caused by problems with signalling or with sensing.

Nerves

The nerves sending signals to our spinal cord and brain can become damaged. Put very simply, the connection is like an electrical cable signal – if there's a fault somewhere along the line the bladder won't receive the message that it needs to be emptied. This can result in different types of incontinence, including urge incontinence, stress incontinence or a mixture of both (see Chapter 5).

Sensors

If the sensors on the bladder wall aren't functioning correctly, someone may feel the need to go to the toilet when the bladder hasn't reached its threshold limit (that is, there may be very little urine in the bladder) and their bladder will contract at the wrong time – this will also give rise to urgency and leaks.

Neurological conditions that affect bladder function

As we have seen, our brain and nervous systems are an integral part of bladder function. Therefore, any damage to the brain and spinal cord in the CNS or other nerves in the peripheral nervous system can result in bladder issues.[27] Conditions such as multiple sclerosis (MS), where there is damage to the covering of nerve cells in the spinal cord and brain, often lead to bladder problems.[28] In fact, reviews of the research show that 80-100% of people with MS have some sort of bladder problem over the course of their illness.[29] This additional set of symptoms can have a major impact on people's lives, with 70% of MS patients saying that bladder dysfunction affected their day-to-day life significantly or moderately. Furthermore, treatment of bladder problems in those with a progressive neurological condition like MS can be complicated, and symptom relief may only be temporary, with the need for regular re-assessment.

Because the spinal cord is an essential part of the central nervous system, damage to it can result in problems with every organ in the body, including the bladder.[30] People with neurological conditions such as spinal cord injury often have both bladder and bowel dysfunction.[31] These secondary health conditions often lead to a bigger impact on life than any other aspect, such as personal background,[32] as they can limit not only day-to-day activities but also social and intimate relationships.[33] Therefore, it's important that these additional illnesses are understood by scientists, doctors and patients in terms of the relationship between the brain and bladder and bowel, and addressed where possible.

Summary and conclusion

In this chapter, we have explored the ways in which the brain and bladder communicate so that we know when the bladder needs to be emptied. Therefore the nervous system is a fundamental part of the way our bodies store and then pass urine, by the use of intricate controlling and coordinating impulses. This is a complex process which we have covered in brief but we hope sufficiently to give some insight into why some treatments for certain bladder complaints don't appear to target the bladder directly.

In the next chapter, we look at an exciting area of research – the gut microbiota – as we have found this is very much involved in bladder health and illness.

Chapter 4

Brain-gut interactions and microbiota (gut and urinary)

*The gut microbiota–brain axis postulates bi-directional
influences between the microbiota residing in the gut and brain
function, including emotional behavior and cognitive function.*
José-Manuel Fernandez-Real and colleagues[34]

This chapter focuses on a very important topic: that of the trillions of micro-organisms in our guts *and* urinary systems. The micro-organisms in our bowels, collectively known as the gut 'microbiota', are incredibly important to our health. Here we explain the ways in which they may get disturbed, contributing to all sorts of different conditions and diseases, including bladder conditions. We briefly talk about the ways in which the brain, gut and microbiota work together. This system (the microbiota) is so important that some scientists say it should be classified as an organ in its own right, just like the kidneys or the pancreas. It's very important not to skip this chapter; although it may sometimes seem a bit technical, it can really help you understand that you can alter your microbiota by not using products which adversely affect it, and providing it with foods which help support its balance and diversity.

The gut microbiota

It may seem strange that we are going to discuss the gut in a book about the bladder but there are good reasons for this. First of all, the bladder and bowel are linked, but more importantly in this chapter, we are interested not in the gut itself but rather the gut microbiota and how this collection of micro-organisms has now been shown to influence a wide range of health issues.

The brain–gut axis (BGA)

In our previous book on irritable bowel syndrome (IBS), we described the communication system called the brain–gut axis (BGA) which controls the gut:

> *The BGA includes the central nervous system (CNS) which consists of the brain and spinal cord, the enteric nervous system (in the gut) and the hypothalamic-pituitary-adrenal system or 'axis' (the HPA). Now, stress of any sort aggravates any illness and is a factor in all illnesses. This is not simply a psychological phenomenon... our bodies deal with stressful events by altering our physiology.*

Arroll and Dancey

For more in-depth reading about this, see the list of references and further reading on page 185.

Stress and the microbiota

Continuous or repeated stress activates the HPA axis and has subsequent effects on your body. We now know that these mechanisms affect the gut. This has been found to be of particular significance to people with IBS and inflammatory bowel disease (IBD), but now we know that the microbiota are linked to all sorts of illnesses.

We know that any sort of stress is likely to lead to altered microbiota. It has been shown that early-life stress alters behaviour, immunity and microbiota in rats.[35] Another study found that stress affected the microbiota of mice.[36] The researchers said that when the stress was repeated over six consecutive 24-hour periods, there was a physiological stress response. That is, the HPA axis was activated, which demonstrated stress. The researchers carrying out this study showed that psychological stressors disrupt the composition of gut microbiota, which of course has important health implications.

The microbiota and the gastrointestinal tract (GIT)

Professor Douglas Drossman, an expert in IBS and IBD who has worked in gastroenterology for many decades, stated that disorders such as IBS are due to 'mucosal immune dysfunction' and abnormalities in gut microbiota. These problems are also relevant to people with bladder conditions.

All of us have trillions of live micro-organisms in our bodies, the vast majority of which live in our guts. The internal lining of the GIT is a large mucosal surface; this surface is semi-permeable, allowing substances such as nutrients to pass through the barrier, but preventing pathogens (things which harm us) getting through. The GIT interacts with the brain and the immune system, ensuring that our immune system is strong, and decreasing the likelihood of us getting infections. We have between 500 and 1000 species of these microbiota, all of which have evolved to live with us in our body. The relationship we have with the microbiota is 'symbiotic' – that is, the microbiota cannot survive without us, and we cannot survive without them: it is a two-way relationship. We give them a place where they can live in the right temperature, and provide them with nutrients, while they help us stay healthy.

'Good' and 'bad' bacteria

All of us play host to different amounts of 'good bacteria' (such asbifidobacteria and lactobacilli) and 'bad bacteria' (such as clostridia) and the majority of these micro-organisms are located in our guts. When we researched the importance of gut microbiota for our last book (on IBS), we found that these micro-organisms played a larger part than we had thought, both in our general health and in IBS in particular. The microbiota develop a tolerance to toxins that normally lead to an immune response in our bodies, so that, over time, we become immune to these toxins so that they don't produce an inflammatory response, which would have led to illness. If the microbiota get out of balance, then this can lead to increased immune activity which can in turn result in low-grade inflammation; this has been found to be the case with IBS.[37] It has become apparent, however, that abnormalities in gut microbiota are associated with many different diseases and conditions, not just IBS.

For instance, disturbances in gut microbiota have been associated with:

- allergies
- anxiety
- asthma
- autism
- Behcet's syndrome
- coeliac disease
- colon cancer
- depression
- diabetes
- endometriosis
- hypertension
- liver disease
- metabolic disease
- ME
- obesity
- Parkinson's disease
- rheumatic diseases.

And most likely UTIs/cystitis.

The microbiota do not work in isolation, but are part of the brain–gut axis.

*The gastrointestinal tract is the primary site of interaction
between the host immune system and microorganisms, both
symbiotic and pathogenic.*

Round & Mazmanian[38]

A unique environment

As we have said, we are born with these trillions of live micro-organisms, which live with us and have evolved with us. However, we don't all have the same composition of microbiota in our guts. Differences in our microbiota after we are born are likely to be due to different feeding patterns in infancy. The composition of our microbiota fluctuates and changes until it becomes more or less stable when we are around three years old.

Different people have different proportions of the various organisms partly due to differences in life experiences, diet, the illnesses and diseases they have, the substances they are exposed to, and the food, antibiotics and drugs they ingest.
Jeremy Nicholson and colleagues say:

*Interactions between the gut microbiota and the host immune
system begin at birth. The microbiota shapes the development
of the immune system, and the immune system in turn shapes
the composition of the microbiota.*[39]

Microbiotic family ties

However, researchers have noted that family members tend to have more similar microbiotic environments than people who are not related to each other. This could be because they tend to have similar diets, but researchers collaborating at different institutions in several countries say that some bacteria are inherited. They say that human genetics shape the microbiotic environment in the gut. This could explain obesity where children of obese parents tend also to be obese. Often, people think obese children might be obese because they are following the dietary habits of their obese parents. Of course, it *might* be that simple. But because we know the microbiotic environment is linked to obesity, it is probably the case that infants share their parents' microbiota.

This cutting-edge research has implications for health:

> *Once the interactions between host genetics and the*
> *microbiome are understood, its manipulation could be*
> *optimized for a given host genome to reduce disease risk.*
>
> Goodrich and colleagues[40]

Working in partnership – the brain and the gut

In 2015, José-Manuel Fernandez-Real and colleagues carried out a study to determine whether the gut microbiota affect brain structure (which can be thought of as the hardware) and brain function (the software – memory, talking, performing calculations). Evidence from animal studies had suggested this was the case, and other studies had found that taking probiotics led to brain changes. This was a very detailed, complex study. The 39 participants were given blood and other laboratory tests and measured on many different dimensions. This included measuring gut microbiota, brain microstructure, brain imaging (MRIs) and cognitive tests. The researchers concluded that the microbiota affect the brain microstructure and that there is 'function crosstalk'. In a biological system, this means that one (or more) components affect other components as a result of communicating with them. The communication is called 'signalling'.

The gut microbiota, then, form part of the brain–gut axis, and there is ongoing, two-way communication between these two organs. In other words, our brain communicates with our gut and gut microbiota, through signalling, working towards maintaining homeostasis (everything in balance). When we are coasting along in life and not under undue pressure, the signalling from the brain to the microbiota causes no issues – in other words, there is balance. But if we are psychologically or emotionally overwhelmed, our guts and the bacteria that reside there also become upset. Furthermore, the composition of the microbiota can be adversely affected by various products, including antibiotics and other medications, which then signal to the brain and can potentially lead to anxiety and depression. In other words, because the brain and gut communicate via signalling, if a person is 'stressed', the other (gut or brain) will in turn become distressed.[41]

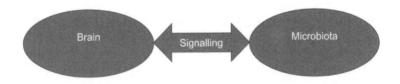

Figure 5: The microbiota–gut–brain axis is made up of the two-way communication, through multiple pathways, between the gut and the brain.[41]

Many antibiotics reduce the 'good' bacteria, with an increase in the 'bad' bacteria. In a review of microbiota in relation to anxiety and depression, Luna and Foster noted that studies showed that stress alone, and antibiotics alone, both reduced the good bacteria in the gut.[42] However, the combination of stress and antibiotics together gave an even greater reduction in good bacteria than would have been expected. Although researchers have known for a long time that stress affects the gastrointestinal tract, it is only very recently that they have realised that stress affects the microbiota.

Of note to those of us with bladder infections: stress can influence the outcome of bacterial infection, because gut bacteria react to the release of stress-related neurochemicals we produce when we are stressed.

It is not just antibiotics that cause us problems; the microbiota are adversely affected by other substances such as:

- artificial sweeteners
- laxatives
- other medications

... and, and no doubt other products which have not yet been researched.

How can we nurture the gut microbiota?

Knowing the importance of the gut microbiota to disease processes, and the ways in which their composition can be altered, it's possible for us to improve our health by choosing not to use substances which adversely affect them, and by eating foods which might improve their composition (see Chapter 10, page 115).

Research shows that people with IBS often show abnormal amounts of bad bacteria and/or a restricted number of microbiotic species. What we need, it seems, is good *diversity* of these micro-organisms. We know that pre- and pro-biotics, and certain foods and drinks, are better at helping with IBS symptoms than placebo. The work with people with IBS shows that it is possible to change the composition of our microbiota, which then helps bring our microbiota back into balance.

Urinary microbiota

We know far less about urinary microbiota, because the research relating to this is very recent. It had been thought for decades that the bladder was a sterile environment. However, recent research has shown that micro-organisms also reside in the bladder. Researchers showed that women with urinary urgency incontinence had vastly different urinary microbiota from women without the condition. Nienhouse and colleagues found that people with urinary incontinence had increased Gardnerella (bad bacteria) and decreased Lactobacilli (good bacteria) compared with people without incontinence.[43] Linda Brubaker and Alan Wolfe carried out a review of the urinary microbiota. They say that the female urinary microbiota (FUM)

> *is likely to modify the diagnosis, prevention and treatment of adult women with urinary disorders.*
>
> Brubaker and Wolfe[44]

As with micro-organisms in the gut, different women have differing compositions relating to their FUM. The challenge now is to determine how to restore the FUM to a healthy state, which will in turn give symptom relief to women.

Another study studied 25 men with chronic prostatitis (CP) or chronic pelvic pain (CPPS) and 25 men without these illnesses.[45] The researchers found people with CP/CPPS had a different microbiotic environment from the other men.

A study published in July 2016 said that a shift in the urinary microbiota might play a part in urgency urinary incontinence (UUI).[46] First, the researchers identified that microbiota existed in the bladders of both healthy controls (women without UUI) and women with UUI. They found that the urinary microbiota played an important part in UUI, and that the loss of microbial diversity might be associated with more severe UUI. Their studies provided evidence that overactive bladder syndrome (OAB) symptoms, including UUI, could be influenced by alterations in the urinary microbiotic environment.

The team working at Loyola University Chicago Health Sciences Division carried out many research projects in infectious diseases and immunology, including work on urinary microbiota. They say that there is evidence for the existence of a community of bacteria that *protect* individuals against UTIs.

This research is expected to lead to new treatments for OAB and people with UTIs/cystitis, but this will take some time.

Summary and conclusion

Here we have looked at a new and emerging area of research – that of the microbiota. Increasingly, scientists and doctors are becoming aware of the important part our microbiotic colonies play in our health and wellbeing. In the future, we may find that treatments are targeted at this area for many conditions, including bladder illness.

In the next chapter, we begin looking at some of these bladder conditions and the symptoms of bladder dysfunction.

Chapter 5

Urinary incontinence, overactivity and retention

When I was a student I had an interest in incontinence but as an undergrad we hardly get any training at all, most courses even now only include about two hours' training, and it's the same with medics and nurses – there's hardly anything. But after I had my family I went back to the subject as it's common but yet so fixable – I remembered that from 20 years earlier and yet nobody was speaking about it. I was really interested in incontinence stuff because if I was gonna spend my time in working with somebody, it's good to have as big an impact as possible for job satisfaction.

Elaine Miller, physiotherapist and comedian

In this chapter, we start by describing the different types of urinary incontinence that people experience. Incontinence can be a diagnosis of its own or a symptom of another problem, often an overactive bladder. Overactive bladder syndrome (OAB) can be due to miscommunication between the bladder and brain, which is why we needed to explore this relationship in Chapter 3. Finally, we discuss not being able to pass urine (known as bladder retention) which can also lead to incontinence. All of these symptoms can have a major impact on the way people live their lives and the enjoyment of day-to-day activities. And as everyone with bladder problems just wants to know how to get better, Chapters 9–15 use the knowledge covered here to discuss a range of treatments that help people to regain bladder control once again. As Elaine says above, incontinence is common yet fixable, so you needn't live with these distressing symptoms.

Incontinence

Being incontinent is extremely upsetting. Most of us wouldn't leave the house at all if we thought we might 'have an accident' as there is a great deal of stigma and embarrassment attached to the inability to control our bladder (discussed in Chapter 1). Urinary incontinence is still seen as taboo. Articles in the media openly talk about mental health as being the 'last taboo' but research shows that incontinence is viewed as more shameful than depression or cancer.[47] This is one reason why many people do not go to their doctors and ask for help, but rather try to cope as best they can on their own. Even when people see medical professionals for other health problems, they often feel unable to discuss their incontinence,[48] but bladder issues and incontinence aren't, in any way, a personal failing even if our current culture leads us to feel that way.

Types of incontinence

Incontinence comes in many forms. To find the best treatment it's important to understand which type or types you may have. These are:
- stress incontinence
- urge incontinence
- overflow incontinence
- total incontinence
- functional incontinence.

Stress incontinence

The word stress here isn't referring to 'being stressed' or anxious, rather that the bladder is under more pressure than it can handle. If we think again about the bladder as a balloon, if the tie on the balloon is not tight enough and someone suddenly squeezes the full, or partially full, balloon, the water inside will gush out. This is what happens in stress incontinence, usually because the pelvic floor muscles or sphincters muscles (Chapter 3, page 33) are weak or damaged. Back to the balloon analogy – the internal pressure of a cough, sneeze or laugh can be thought of as the abrupt high-pressure squeezing of the balloon/bladder which causes urine to leak out. Exercise can also trigger stress incontinence – for some people something as simple as a walk or lifting a heavy object can lead to 'an accident'.[49] Stress incontinence can impact a person's life in many ways, including taking part in fun activities, as Tanya explains:

> It affects me in the choices I make in my personal life so when work colleagues suggested going trampolining as a night out, my first thought was, 'Oh god I can't do that, I might wet myself, and how embarrassing would that be!' I also worry when I feel like I'm going to sneeze or cough as I have to tense and concentrate hard to not 'leak'! This can also be said for uncontrollable laughter!
>
> *Tanya*

What causes stress incontinence?

Because stress incontinence is linked to weakening of the pelvic floor muscles, it may start after childbirth, particularly if the birth was natural (vaginal birth) rather than by caesarean section. Pelvic floor muscles can also be affected by the bodily changes during the menopause; however, as with all muscles, the pelvic floor can be strengthened with targeted exercises (see Chapter 9). Another cause of stress incontinence specifically in women is the possible injury to the bladder during surgical removal of the womb (hysterectomy). This is because the bladder sits below the womb and can be injured during surgery.

Stress incontinence is most common in pregnant women – in studies carried out around the world, on average 40% of women have stress incontinence either during or after pregnancy.[50] During pregnancy, the increasing weight of the unborn baby puts more and more pressure on the pelvic floor muscles, which may cause leakage. As in the menopause, changing hormones too can affect both the pelvic floor[51] and the function of the sphincter.[52] Furthermore, the breakdown of collagen during pregnancy has also been suggested as a reason for stress incontinence as women with less overall collagen have been shown to be more likely to suffer from stress incontinence.[53] Collagen is a substance which gives our connective tissues their tensile strength and elasticity. This may be why people with Ehlers-Danlos syndrome (a genetic condition which affects the production of collagen) often have urinary issues such as stress incontinence.[54]

In men, surgery to remove the prostate gland can trigger stress incontinence. In both men and women, being overweight or obese may put undue pressure on the bladder. Neurological conditions that affect the central nervous system (such as multiple sclerosis and Parkinson's disease) can also bring about this type of incontinence. When neurological conditions affect the bladder like this, the symptoms are often said to be due to a 'neurogenic bladder', in which the messages between the brain–bladder have been interrupted (Chapter 3).

He diagnosed me with neurogenic bladder. He said that it could be that my bladder is sending wrong signals to my brain, or my brain is sending wrong signals to my bladder. As a baby I had small strokes; I was born two months premature. I am also a

twin. My brother and I had to be reanimated after our hearts
stopped and we stopped breathing. The urologist said that the
lack of the oxygen to the brain, and the strokes we suffered are
most likely the cause of the bladder problems I experience.

Martine

Urge incontinence

Urinary urgency, or urge incontinence, is the overwhelming
need to find a toilet as soon as the initial sensation of needing to
wee starts. As we age, our bladders may seem to have a mind of
their own and can demand we go to the toilet more frequently
than we used to, and/or give us little warning that we need to
go. This urgency can lead to accidents either during the day or
at night. Many people have mixed stress and urge incontinence,
which can both be thought of as problems with the storage phase
of micturition (see Chapter 3, page 30).

What causes urge incontinence?

Unsurprisingly, what we drink can affect our bladder. Caffeine is
both a stimulant and a diuretic – that is, it increases the production
of urine. While moderate amounts of caffeinated drinks don't
seem to result in urge incontinence, drinking numerous cups of
coffee, tea or other caffeine-containing drinks does increase the
likelihood of needing to go to the toilet urgently and frequently.[55]
Research in those with urge incontinence has demonstrated that
reducing caffeine intake to less than 100 mg per day (which
equates to about four cups of tea or a single cup of coffee) can
help people not only to feel less sudden need to urinate, but also
actually go to the toilet less often.[56] However, not everyone finds
caffeinated drinks a problem – see Chapter 10 for more about
what foods and drinks are 'bladder friendly'.

On the other hand, drinking too little can also lead to urge incontinence as highly concentrated urine may irritate the bladder wall. Infections such as cystitis (see Chapter 6, page 58), constipation, bladder tumours, medications (e.g. diuretics, medicines for high blood pressure, some antidepressants and sleeping pills) and neurological conditions (as above) can be the reason for this type of incontinence. However, urgency can also be due to miscommunication between the brain and the bladder where the detrusor muscle (page 33) contracts too much, making you feel as if your bladder is full and needs to be emptied right away when in fact it doesn't. When this is the case, and often when there is no clear reason for symptoms, bladder urgency and frequency are labelled as 'overactive bladder syndrome'.

Overactive bladder syndrome (OAB)

As we have said, sometimes people with urge incontinence will be diagnosed with overactive bladder syndrome (or OAB), but not everyone with OAB will leak urine. However, the urgent and immediate need to go to the toilet is characteristic of OAB. Other symptoms of OAB are:

- needing to pass urine more than eight times a day (frequency)
- at night-time, needing to leave bed to get up to go to the toilet on more than one occasion (nocturia)
- wetting the bed (nocturnal enuresis)
- leaking urine during sexual intercourse in women (coital incontinence).

Whilst all of these symptoms are upsetting, embarrassing and difficult to talk about, it is perhaps the last that is given least attention and discussion. However, coital incontinence is not uncommon in women with bladder problems. One study of 633 women seeking help for OAB in a gynaecology clinic found more than a third leaked urine during sex.[57] Symptoms such as coital incontinence directly affect how often women with OAB want to have sex,[58] which of course can push couples apart, especially if they find bladder issues too hard to talk about. Considering that estimates of OAB in women are 17% (lower for men, at about 10%),[59] these problems are hidden behind closed doors but affect people's quality of life significantly. Many people suffer in silence because they feel embarrassed to talk to their GP, think that there is no treatment, or think it's just that they are getting old. However, there are treatments which can help.

What causes OAB?

OAB is where the detrusor muscle layer of the bladder contracts too much and when the bladder isn't necessarily full.[60] The causes of OAB are similar to those of urge incontinence and as such, some doctors and researchers use these terms inter-changeably. However, someone with OAB may not be incontinent, as they may be able to get to a toilet in time.[61] And whilst OAB may be triggered by an infection, too many caffeinated drinks, an obstruction, medicines or a neurological condition, this won't happen in everyone. The most common explanation for OAB is that the bladder somehow becomes more sensitive or more easily irritated, by caffeine for instance. But why some people's bladders become sensitive and others do not is still under debate. Nevertheless, there are numerous ways to treat an OAB, which we explore in Chapters 9 to 15.

Overflow incontinence

Overflow incontinence is pretty much what it sounds like – the amount of urine builds up in the bladder and overflows, or leaks out. This is because in people with overflow incontinence, the bladder doesn't completely empty when going to the toilet (known as urinary retention). There may be difficulty in passing water initially, and a weak and inconsistent flow once it starts. Because there's still some wee left in the bladder, it fills more quickly and there's less room, meaning leaks can happen. If we think of stress and urge incontinence as issues to do with the storage phase of micturition, then overflow incontinence is a problem of the voiding phase (Chapter 3, page 30).

> At 21 my condition became worse. I could not fully void my bladder, I had pressure, when I had to hold the larger amount of fluid I felt like my bladder was going to burst, I could barely walk from the pain of a full bladder. I suffered like this for a few years until I finally talked to my father about it, and we went to see a urologist and I explained my symptoms.
>
> *Martine*

What causes overflow incontinence?

Constipation may be one explanation for overflow incontinence so if you are having trouble passing stools (poo), discuss this with your doctor and/or pharmacist as there are many over-the-counter and effective remedies for constipation (page 128). Bladder stones may also cause a blockage that prevents complete urination. In men, an enlarged prostate gland may also be causing problems with bladder voiding. Yet again, neurological conditions or damage to the central nervous system (such as spinal cord injury) are associated with inadequate emptying of the bladder. People who have diabetes may also develop a condition known as 'diabetic bladder dysfunction', which can lead to both storage and voiding problems.[62]

The detrusor muscles may also contribute to overflow incontinence. This is because the bladder itself can become stretched if the detrusor muscles do not fully contract and push out the full volume of urine in the bladder. Hence, healthy and unimpeded communication between the bladder and brain is important for good bladder control.

Trauma within the body, such as during surgical procedures and giving birth, can also lead to urine retention that may result in overflow incontinence. This can occur when the bladder itself does not appear to be damaged and is often overlooked by healthcare professionals, especially in older people.[63] Urine retention can be very distressing, as Hannah's case below describes.

Hannah's story of postpartum urinary retention

The day after my son was born and before I was discharged from hospital, the midwife wanted me to have a wee. To my dismay, I just couldn't go. I pushed and pushed until something came out, but it was clear something wasn't right. The midwife used a bladder scanner and commented that I was retaining a lot of urine, but because I had managed to wee a bit she let me go home. After that, weeing was a nightmare! I continued to suffer and to push and squeeze to get any urine out. Six days after the birth, I saw my GP who organised for me to go back to hospital.

So, on Day 7 I went back to the postnatal ward and a midwife fitted a catheter, and it had a bag that was attached to my leg to collect the urine. The plan was to have that for a couple of days in order to rest my bladder. I really hated that bag! On Day 9, I went back to have it removed to see if I could void my bladder. I couldn't get a single drop of wee out and I was utterly beside myself. However, the midwife told me that she had dealt previously with ladies who had suffered with postpartum urinary retention and all of them had regained the ability to wee, although the recovery time was different for each. I felt such relief to hear this. She explained that sometimes the trauma of labour can make the bladder go into shock. She fitted me with another catheter but this one had no bag, instead it had a valve which I opened every four hours to empty my bladder. The idea was to teach my bladder to fill up and then empty. I had this catheter for about a week. Although it was better than having a bag, I found it very uncomfortable, particularly when I was standing up and walking, I could feel it inside me.

On Day 15, I was back on the postnatal ward and had the catheter removed so I could try and void my bladder again. I was terrified. What if I couldn't wee after this? I drank a load of water and waited. Eventually I had a sensation of fullness (although the sensation was not as strong as it was before I gave birth) so I went off to the bathroom. And I couldn't go. I tried running the taps, waiting, reading a magazine to relax... nothing. Again, I burst into tears. After a while I could get something out when I squeezed and pushed, but it hurt to do this and I was advised not to do so anyway. The bladder scanner unsurprisingly revealed I was retaining a lot of urine. The next step was self-catheterisation...

The advice was to try and wee on my own, and then to use a catheter. To begin with I couldn't wee on my own at all, but after four or five days of using the catheters, I started to be able to wee a little. What a feeling! The sensation, however, was entirely different to before I had my baby. It's hard to explain but when the urine started to flow, there wasn't really much feeling in my wee hole and it felt like the wee was coming out in a different location to where it used to (which of course it wasn't because, as far as I know, it was in the same place!). Also, the flow was really slow and if I tried to stop mid-flow then there was no chance of being able to finish off the wee. Annoyingly, after a couple of days of really feeling like I was making progress, I couldn't wee on my own anymore. Although I was upset, I took comfort in the fact that other ladies on this thread had experienced this, that there were good days followed by bad days, but these bad days were followed by good days.

Six weeks on I can wee on my own without having to use a catheter (and without needing to have a bath!). There were days when I honestly thought that this would never happen. As my episiotomy/tear has healed, the ability to wee has been improving. However, the sensation is different to how it used to be, although it is getting stronger each day. Last week it took a few goes to completely empty my bladder on occasion – by this I mean that I could void most of my bladder, then a few seconds or minutes later I needed to wee a little bit more. However, this week I feel that I can get it all out in one go. The physiotherapist I have been seeing at the hospital (for advice about pelvic floor exercises since this might help the bladder problem) suggested leaning my body forward or to the side towards the end of the wee to help encourage the last drops out, and absolutely not to push as this works against pelvic floor muscles. She also suggested I should stand up after a wee, squeeze the pelvic floor muscles, relax them and then sit back on the toilet to help the last drops come out.

Finally, I don't give much time to thinking about weeing!

Hannah

Total incontinence

Total urinary incontinence is when the bladder is unable to hold urine at all – even small amounts. This total loss of urinary control means that wee leaks constantly, whether the person has gone to the toilet or not.

What causes total incontinence?

Bladder abnormalities from birth may lead to total incontinence. Spinal cord injury can completely interrupt bladder–brain communication, as can other neurological conditions. In women, a small opening can develop between the bladder and vagina known as a fistula, causing unconscious and continual leakage from this hole.

Functional incontinence

Functional incontinence differs from the types described above as someone with this type of urinary problem will be fully aware that they need to urinate, but other conditions will make it difficult to find a toilet in time. Also for some people environmental factors such as toilets that are challenging to access and use, low toilet seats that are hard to get up from and poor lighting can lead to functional incontinence.

What causes functional incontinence?

People who have mobility difficulties, dementia, very poor eyesight, poor dexterity, severe mental health issues may experience functional incontinence.

Summary and conclusion

In this chapter, we've looked at different types of incontinence and discussed how these relate to urinary retention and OAB. Incontinence can have a significant impact on people's lives as it often leads to embarrassment and feelings of shame. However, there are many treatment options which we will outline later in this book – it may take a combination of medicine, diet and exercise but many people do overcome bladder problems. In the next chapter, we will look in more detail at bladder (urinary tract) infection, which is more commonly called cystitis. We'll also discuss a condition that has the same symptoms as an infection but where tests come back negative. This condition is called interstitial cystitis or painful bladder syndrome and shares some of the symptoms of OAB, which is why these conditions are often difficult to diagnose.

Chapter 6

Cystitis and interstitial cystitis

In this chapter, we continue looking at bladder illness, starting with a common infection that is easily identified and treated – cystitis. Then we explore a condition that has the same symptoms, but isn't due to bacterial infection – interstitial cystitis (amongst other names). Even though these conditions have similar names, they can differ substantially in the length of time it takes to receive a diagnosis, how they affect daily life and the treatments available. While cystitis is a condition that sometimes can either be self-treated or remedied with a one-off visit to a GP, interstitial cystitis can take many years to diagnose as there is no definitive understanding of its cause.

Cystitis/urinary tract infection (UTI)

Cystitis, also called urinary tract infection (UTI), is a very common bladder issue occurring 150 million times worldwide every year. In fact, cystitis is one of the most common complaints seen by GPs and almost half of the world population will experience a cystitis during their lives.[64]

> On becoming a teenager, I was often diagnosed as
> having cystitis, but I cannot remember many urine samples
> being tested. I was just given antibiotics routinely, as a matter of
> course. I do know that I suffered cystitis symptoms quite often,

which made things worse with regard to how often I needed to go to the toilet.

Sharon

What causes cystitis?

Cystitis is normally caused by bacteria that enter the bladder via the urethra. Because women have shorter urethras, this type of infection is more common in women than men, but anyone (including children) can suffer from it.

What are the symptoms of cystitis?

It was previously thought that urine is bacteria-free and that the presence of bacteria causes infection and inflammation. However, we now know that the bladder and urinary tract are not sterile and therefore urine isn't either. Like the gut, there are good bacteria that live in the bladder which protect against infection. Therefore, it's not simply the presence of any or all bacteria that results in an infection – rather, if the urinary microbiota get out of balance, then infection can take over, which may give you some unpleasant and painful symptoms. These can include:

- needing to wee urgently
- feeling the need to wee more often than usual but often only being able to pass small amounts of urine
- experiencing pain, or a burning or stinging sensation when passing urine
- pain in the lower part of the stomach;
- a general feeling of being unwell – i.e. achy and tired
- passing urine that is darker in colour than is normal for you and sometime with an unusual or strong odour
- blood in the urine.

Adults don't normally have a raised temperature with cystitis (over 38°C or 100.4°F) so a temperature and/or pain in the lower back or sides might be a kidney infection and this should be investigated by a doctor.

How is cystitis treated?

People recognise that an urgent need to pee, as well as a pain or burning sensation when they do so, is indicative of cystitis, and that they need to see a doctor. However, cystitis can resolve itself with some self-help measures and may not need a course of antibiotics. These include:

- drinking water or very weak tea to flush out your system
- using a hot water bottle if you have pain in the lower stomach
- using Canesten oasis/Cymalon sachets (sodium citrate) or Cymalon liquid/Cystopurin (potassium citrate), which make urine less acidic and, purportedly, a less hospitable place for bacteria to multiply
- taking over-the-counter pain medication, such as paracetamol or ibuprofen (though bear in mind the latter can cause constipation in some people – check with the chemist if you're worried about any of the side effects listed in the information leaflet)
- avoiding sexual intercourse until the symptoms have completely resolved.

If your symptoms do not go away or if you are feeling very unwell and have a fever, consult your GP who may ask you for a urine sample and s/he will do a dipstick test to see if there are signs of any abnormalities in your urine. These can include evidence of blood, proteins, nitrates and white blood cells (leucocytes). If your doctor sees a positive dipstick result you may be prescribed antibiotics and the sample may also be sent to the lab to ensure the type of antibiotics that you are given will rid you of the infection. If you have repeated infections, it's important to have your urine samples sent to a lab because you may be not suffering from bacterial infection but rather your bladder may be inflamed without the presence of bacteria – this is known as interstitial cystitis (page 64).

> I had cystitis when I was away from home for two weeks. When I went to the chemist and explained the situation, I was refused any medicine; they said I had to go to a doctor. Unfortunately, this was not possible because the pain when urinating was almost unbearable – I therefore went to a different chemist and said that my girlfriend had the condition.
>
> The sensation was like burning liquid when passing fluid and it came in short bursts because it was too painful to pass in one and my body kept stopping it. Once it got moving it really was incredibly painful and the smell I remember being acrid and very different to when passing normally. At the end of passing it felt like the tubes were closed up and both sharp and dull pains were there for a few minutes – it was like having everything squeezed very painfully. No matter when, during having the condition, I always felt like I needed to pee and there was always a dull ache just below my stomach, I guess where my bladder is. I've only had this condition once and I hope I never get it again because passing what felt like razorblades is not a nice experience.
>
> *Rob*

How do I prevent cystitis?

As mentioned above, women have a shorter urethra than men and this is positioned closer to the back passage (anus), offering more opportunities for bacteria from the back passage to migrate. Because of this, toilet habits are important for women who experience repeated episodes of cystitis. To prevent spreading

---

Does cranberry juice 'cure' cystitis?

Cystitis usually goes away by itself – what doctors would call 'self-limiting' – but these infections can recur, which is very frustrating for anyone who has numerous episodes. If there is a bacterial infection that shows up on the dipstick or lab tests, antibiotics will get rid of the underlying bacterial infection and symptoms will disappear. However, in people who have frequent cystitis, the bacteria can become resistant to the medication. Antibiotic resistance is actually becoming a global problem and doctors are encouraged to limit how many prescriptions they give out in case this increases; bacterial resistance to antibiotics would be a very serious problem considering some infections are life-threatening (e.g. pneumonia, septicaemia, bacterial meningitis).[64A] Also, as mentioned in Chapter 4, antibiotics can disrupt the gut microbiota which can then negatively affect our overall health. Therefore, doctors and researchers are always looking for alternative ways to prevent and treat illnesses like cystitis without using antibiotics. Many people say that drinking cranberry juice or using cranberry supplements helps to control persistent bouts of cystitis. The theory behind this is that cranberries contain a substance that stops bacteria from adhering to the bladder wall, which will then counteract an infection. A systematic review which looked at all the scientific studies available on cranberries (juice, tablets and capsules) showed that using this fruit was better at preventing infections than doing nothing but that cranberries weren't better at preventing cystitis than taking prophylactic antibiotics.[64B] So if you do suffer from frequent cystitis, investing in cranberry products may not be worthwhile.

---

bacteria it's best to dry yourself from the front to back – that is, wiping towards the anus rather than away from it. This often seems counter-intuitive as girls are usually taught the other way round but it is an easy habit to break. Other ways to discourage cystitis are (for women):

- drink plenty of water every day to ensure that the bladder is flushed regularly and thoroughly

- sit leaning back rather than bending forward when passing urine as this will help the bladder empty fully
- urinate before and after sexual intercourse
- don't go for long periods of time without passing urine; try to go at least once every couple of hours.

Men who experience a UTI/cystitis should discuss this with their doctors as this could be a sign of an enlarged prostate, infection in the prostate (prostatitis), and or an infection in the urethra (urethritis).

Pregnant women who have UTI/cystitis symptoms should always consult their doctor.

Antibiotics – to use or not to use?
Antibiotics are truly one of the great medical advances of our times, saving countless lives and leading to the near eradication of some deadly diseases in developed countries. However, as Uncle Ben says to Peter Parker in Spiderman, 'With great power comes great responsibility'.

Overuse of antibiotics is now known to lead to antibiotic resistance. This is when bacteria alter and so are no longer affected by the drug – they are clever really. For the individual host (i.e. the patient), this is a big problem as the antibiotics simply won't work anymore. So there is now a drive for doctors to prescribe antibiotics only when absolutely necessary as you never know when you might really need them – for example, for life-threatening bloodstream infections and pneumonia. Furthermore, crucial life-saving treatments, such chemotherapy, and procedures such organ transplant, could lead to death if we didn't have effective ways to prevent infection. Even routine operations such as caesareans and hip replacements become high-risk if infection cannot be controlled.

While a short course of antibiotics may successfully treat a single bacterial infection of the urinary tract, this won't prevent repeated infections. Although some people may be treated with low-dose prophylactic (preventative) antibiotics,

---

this doesn't work for everyone. We also now know that these drugs can play havoc with our microbiota, destroying both the good and bad bacteria in our guts. Therefore, antibiotic use can harm this important part of our immune system and lead to conditions such as IBS (in those predisposed to the condition). Therefore, trying all non-drug approaches such as dietary changes and fluid intake might help to avoid recurrent cystitis.

Interstitial cystitis (IC)

Some people have the symptoms of cystitis, but when the doctor tests the urine sample, there are no signs of an infection. This can be very frustrating for people as they might feel that doctors don't believe them when they are in extreme discomfort. Interstitial cystitis (IC), 'painful bladder syndrome' or sometimes 'chronic bladder inflammation', is a chronic illness where the bladder wall becomes inflamed on a long-term basis. This is an awfully painful condition, where antibiotics are often not effective as there is not a bacterial infection of the bladder, even if it feels like there is one. No one knows for sure what causes IC and people can be undiagnosed or misdiagnosed (often with overactive bladder – Chapter 5, page 51) for many years.

I couldn't even tell you when I first saw the doctor about my bladder but definitely as a teenager – but I don't know exactly when. All the appointments are a bit of a blur now. I had so many 'infections' as a teenager that I got used to the drill pretty quickly. I also started trying things to help then, like not wearing tights and drinking cranberry juice. I still had lots of infections or bouts of cystitis. Back then sometimes it would go away with the chemist's sachets but later the infections or interstitial cystitis was far too bad not to go to the GP and I became very scared when I started experiencing pain, the need to wee and bloating (I get very bloated with a UTI). I wasn't referred to a specialist until my mid or late 20s and even then I saw two, one who was absolutely awful and subjected me to intimate investigations in front of medical students (I didn't realise at the time I could refuse) and the other gave me a bladder diet which did help a bit. Then I saw another who was useless and just gave pills for overactivity, before I finally saw a good one who knew something about IC – that was then in my 30s. So for me getting a diagnosis wasn't easy and I have to say that the NHS was useless – if only they'd taken me seriously at the start maybe I wouldn't have had decades of hell. I try not to think about it now as it makes me too upset.

Sarah

Is IC the same as OAB?

As Sarah mentioned above, sometimes IC can be confused with OAB. This is because many of the symptoms are the same in both conditions. Specialist doctors Scott MacDiarmid and Peter Sand suggest that there is an overlap between symptoms, such as needing to wee urgently and frequently and also having to go to the toilet at night-time, but other symptoms can differentiate the two conditions.[65] While those with OAB suffer from leaks, incontinence is less common in IC. On the other hand, pelvic pain and pain during sex (dyspareunia) are more common in IC than OAB. It is possible to have both conditions at the same time, but if, like Sarah, you feel the diagnosis you've been given is wrong and the treatment isn't working, speak again to your doctor to make sure you have the correct diagnosis.

How common is IC?

Invisible illnesses are often under- or misdiagnosed. Because of the embarrassing nature of these symptoms, people often don't talk about them – so you may have this condition and feel that it's very rare, but actually it isn't as uncommon as we might think. The prevalence of IC may be as high as one in 4.5 women.[66] This condition is much more common in women than men; about 90% of those with IC will be women.

What causes IC?

IC is an example of a contested or medically unexplained disorder (MUD – as in 'as clear as mud' as we like to say!). When a condition is contested, different scientists and doctors will have differing opinions on why people have symptoms – some can be quite unhelpful (but we hope not so often these days), saying things such as 'There's nothing wrong' or 'It's just psychological', whereas others form views based on new research findings, such as links to the microbiota (Chapter 4). However, it may be that many of the explanations are correct, and that different people have different causes for their condition. Whereas it seems perfectly reasonable to accept that diseases such as cancer can arise from a set of risk factors, all of which contribute to the development of such an illness, there is often more reluctance to view contested disorders in this way. Other MUDs include fibromyalgia, chronic fatigue syndrome/ myalgic encephalomyelitis (CFS/ME) and irritable bowel syndrome (IBS). Interestingly, people with one of these conditions often have another, so those with CFS/ME often have IC as well. Below we explore first some of the proposed causes of IC and also why it should not be surprising that some people have more than one condition where the cause isn't known.

Inflammation

Some people with IC have clear signs of inflammation on their bladder lining in the form of tiny haemorrhages (glomerulations) which look a little like starburst on the inside of the bladder. However, not everyone with the symptoms of IC have these noticeable signs of inflammation so we cannot simply say that IC is an 'inflamed bladder'. However, there is evidence of an inflammatory response in the studies that have looked at cells called 'mast cells'. Mast cells are a type of white blood cell that originate from our bone marrow, which are found in most of our bodily tissues, particularly the skin, airways and intestines as these interact with the outside environment.[67] This interaction allows mast cells to recognise pathogens (such as harmful bacteria or viruses) and quickly mount an immune response. Studies have shown mast cell activation in the bladder wall lining and also detrusor muscle (see page 33) in patients with IC.[68] However, because mast cell activation indicates not only an immune response but can also be a sign of an allergic or autoimmune response, the increased numbers of mast cells simply tells us there is a response going on in the bladder – but not *why*.

'Leaky' bladder

You may have heard the term 'leaky gut' in relation to conditions such as IBS. In Chapter 4, we discussed the mucous membranes (mucosa) that are associated with our internal organs. The bladder also has an internal mucosal membrane which protects it from substances in urine. The mucosa is usually very difficult to penetrate, but if this layer is damaged then substances such as potassium can pass through to the bladder lining, irritating it.[69]

In people without bladder conditions, the high levels of potassium in urine cause no symptoms, but research has shown in those with IC the protective mucosa may have become 'leaky' (or permeable).[70] This means that the tight, close-knit structure of the mucosa has loosened, allowing potassium to spread to the bladder tissue, triggering pain and urgency. If we think of the mucosa as a gauze bandage, its structure is like a weave to allow air to a wound but prevent any bits of dirt or irritants entering the wound itself. If this bandage gets damaged somehow, and the weave texture starts to slacken, the wound will no longer be protected as bigger, more damaging irritants can come into contact with the wound. In the case of the bladder, if the mucosa becomes more permeable (perhaps because of infection or autoimmunity – see below), substances will irritate the bladder and produce symptoms. This theory is very similar to that of the 'leaky gut' that is thought to be involved in IBS.[71]

Neurogenic theory

In addition to inflammation of the bladder wall, there is research that suggests the nerves connected to the bladder may be inflamed.[72] This inflammation could result in miscommunication between nerves carrying messages to the brain from the bladder, and vice versa.

Pelvic floor dysfunction

Other experts think that people with IC have a problem with their pelvic floor muscles, which we use to control urination. These problems include muscular tenderness and issues with the connective tissues of the pelvic floor, hip girdle and abdominal wall. As many as 87% of a group of women with IC in one research study group were shown to have these signs of pelvic floor dysfunction.[73]

Autoimmune theory

Some research suggests that IC is an autoimmune illness where the immune system mistakenly attacks the bladder. People with IC often have other conditions, most commonly allergies and Sjögren's syndrome – in fact, between 40 and 80% of people with IC have allergies and over a quarter (28%) have, or probably have, Sjögren's syndrome.[74] Sjögren's syndrome is an autoimmune illness that causes dry eyes and mouth, and in women vaginal dryness, which can lead to pain during sex. Other symptoms include fatigue, muscle and joint pain and inflammation of blood vessels (known as vasculitis). The co-occurrence of these conditions, a general propensity for allergies and the observation that sometimes treatments taken for allergies relieve the symptoms of IC in some people, suggest that it could also be an autoimmune condition.

Other explanations

It has also been suggested that IC may be a symptom of a more widespread problem, as it's been associated with conditions such as fibromyalgia, chronic fatigue syndrome/myalgic encephalomyelitis (CFS/ME), irritable bowel syndrome (IBS) and lupus. Also, as per Chapter 4, recent scientific research shows that gut microbiota (the good and bad bacteria in our gut) have a lot to do with our health. Gut microbiota are relevant not just to people with IBS and inflammatory bowel disease (IBD), but also to those of us with bladder conditions. This is because many things (such as artificial sweeteners, laxatives, medications and stress) adversely affect the composition of the gut microbiota which can then influence health. Hence, the reason why some people seem to have more than one of these contested conditions could be changes in the gut microbiota and brain–gut axis (see page 33).

Does IC run in families?

Women who have a first-degree relative with IC (their mother, a sister) are more likely to develop this condition than those without this familial link.[75] Twin studies which compare identical ('monozygotic', with identical genetic make-up) twins with non-identical ('dizygotic' – siblings who share a womb) twins have shown that identical twins more frequently both have IC than do non-identical twins.[76] This suggests that there is a hereditary component to IC and that some people may have a genetic predisposition to this condition.

Why is IC so hard to diagnose?

The symptoms of IC are not just very similar to those of UTIs/ cystitis, but also to those of chronic urethral syndrome, overactive bladder syndrome, vulvodynia (a condition in women where there is a feeling of burning and soreness in the vulva but without a skin condition or infection that could explain this discomfort) and endometriosis. Also, it's possible that we can have more than one of these conditions at the same time – for example, IC, chronic pelvic pain *and* endometriosis. In a study of 178 women with chronic pelvic pain, 75% of these patients were found to have endometriosis and 89% were diagnosed with IC.[77] Both conditions were present in 65% of the women in this study, leading the authors to comment that both diagnoses should be considered at the same time in patients who have chronic pelvic pain to avoid unneeded delay in diagnosis and treatment.

However, in everyday medical practice we might receive a diagnosis for one condition and subsequent treatment, but then find some symptoms continue to linger because the co-occurring condition has not been detected. Furthermore, it can be difficult to receive treatment for conditions such as endometriosis – on average it takes 7.5 years from first visiting a doctor to getting the diagnosis, and this is before finding an effective treatment. Some people feel 'fobbed off' with being told they have other conditions like IBS; so, it can take an immense amount of courage and energy to go back time and time again to your doctor if you think you've been misdiagnosed. Many of us, sadly, can have an incredibly frustrating journey to untangle this web of symptoms.

How is IC diagnosed?

Doctors will start with a detailed medical and family history to try and rule out any other conditions that may be the cause of the bladder symptoms; in this sense, the diagnosis of IC can be thought of as a 'diagnosis via exclusion' and some healthcare practitioners stop there. However, if both the doctor and patient want further information or if the diagnosis is unclear, a cystoscopy may be performed[78] (Chapter 8, page 86). When looking at the inside of the bladder during this procedure, it is possible to see whether there are any haemorrhages present. There may also be evidence of scars or lesions called Hunner's ulcers, with low bladder capacity due to tissue stiffening (fibrosis).

Summary and conclusion

In this chapter, we have looked at two conditions which generate almost identical symptoms but one of which (cystitis) is often caused by a bacterial infection while the other (interstitial cystitis – IC) is of unknown origin, or rather there is no consensus as to its precise cause. IC is comparable to conditions such as IBS in that there is a range of research on these conditions that showed different sorts of abnormalities – and in fact some similar findings in terms of mast cells and epithelial permeability. So, as we have previously suggested in our model of IBS, all or some of these mechanisms may be at play in each person with this condition. In this sense, it may take time to find a treatment that works for you. In the next chapter, we look at the condition many of us worry about the most – cancer.

Chapter 7

Bladder cancer

Having cancer, any type of cancer, can be one of our greatest fears. The reasons for this are in some ways obvious – it can be life-threatening and has a big impact on our lives including time off work, hospital visits and not being able to do everyday activities for a time. Cancers are prevalent – half of all people in the UK will be diagnosed with a form of cancer in their lifetime. There are more than 200 types of cancer and sometimes cancer can spread from one part of the body to another. However, importantly, with advances in research and medical practices, survival rates are continually improving. In this chapter, we look at cancer of the bladder and, more specifically, at the aspects of our lives that can make us more at risk of developing bladder cancer.

My mother was 50 when she was diagnosed with bladder cancer. That was in the 1980s when cancer diagnostics and treatment weren't as advanced as they are now. She went to the GP because she noticed blood in her urine and scans showed a cyst in the bladder wall. I remember there was lots of talk about it probably being benign and I remember she had radiotherapy and surgery to remove it – I'm not sure which order they came in. I think everyone thought the problem had gone away, but about a year later a follow-up scan revealed a shadow on her liver and Mum was told the cancer had spread and there was nothing they could do. She died three months later. I remember being furious that she hadn't opted to have her entire bladder removed the year before instead of just the cyst and I have often thought since how I'd much rather have had another decade with my mother with a catheter bag than no mother at all. I was 21 when she died, my brother was 22 and my sister just 19.

Everyone said how rare bladder cancer was and how unusual it was for her to get it, but I read something about the possible link with dyes and chemicals. Mum was a cake decorator by trade and would spend hours piping exquisite miniature roses out of coloured icing. If she stopped to chat, the piping tube would temporarily block with dry icing and she'd suck the end, just briefly, to get the icing flowing again. I can only assume that her consumption of food colouring accumulated over the years, causing a toxic build-up that irritated her bladder lining.

I am hugely relieved to have learned that bladder cancer doesn't appear to have the hereditary links of some other cancers, but it doesn't stop me being paranoid. In my 20s, I started getting cystitis regularly. The first time I peed blood I have to confess I was absolutely terrified.

After a year of near constant antibiotics and fear I discovered that the contraceptive cap (diaphragm) I was using at the time was irritating my bladder wall, and the spermicidal jelly you have to use with it was mucking about with my body's natural defence mechanisms. The attacks stopped when my boyfriend dumped me!

I have since been advised to be vigilant and see my GP if I spot blood in my urine. I'm pretty sure they'd be able to treat my mother's liver cancer now, or at least slow its progression to give her longer with her family. But I'd opt to have my bladder removed in a heartbeat and crochet a natty catheter bag out of high fashion yarn rather than risk the cancer spreading to other organs.

Lucy

How is bladder cancer diagnosed?

Diagnosis of bladder cancer starts with a full personal and family history – your doctor may also ask you about some aspects of your life, for instance if you smoke, in order to weigh up your risk factors (see below).[79] Then you may be asked to provide a urine sample to see if there are any abnormalities, such as blood, bacteria or other substances in your urine. A physical examination of the rectum and/or vagina may also be carried out by your GP (to investigate any lumps that can be a result of bladder cancer) before s/he decides whether to refer you to a specialist urologist. Once within the urology department of a hospital, the next step is to have a cystoscopy (Chapter 8, page 86). Imaging investigations such as CT or MRI scans may also be ordered if the consultant feels it is necessary.

Who gets bladder cancer?

Bladder cancer affects the over-60s more frequently than younger people, with two-thirds of people diagnosed with bladder cancer aged over 65.[80] In fact, it is quite rare in those under 40 years of age. Men are more likely to be diagnosed with bladder cancer than women, possibly due to the higher proportion of men that smoke and the places they traditionally work (see risk factors below).

How common is bladder cancer?

Bladder cancer isn't one of the most common types of cancer – cancer of the breast, prostate, lung and bowel are the most frequently occurring kinds of cancer and just these four account for more than half of all new diagnoses in the UK (53%).[81] Bladder cancer is the 10th most commonly occurring cancer, but only accounts for 3% of new cases each year. The good news is that the number of people who experience bladder cancer is actually falling – since the early 1990s we've seen the incidence of bladder cancer drop by 38%. The decline has been greater in men (42%) than women (36%). This may be due to a reduction in smoking over this time period as smoking is the biggest 'risk factor' for bladder cancer. Statisticians predict that bladder cancer rates will continue to fall in the future.

What are the survival rates for bladder cancer?

As with others forms of cancer, survival rates are dependent on the stage of cancer. For **Stage 1** bladder cancer, where cancerous cells have started to grow beneath the bladder lining, and so into connective tissues, nine out 10 people survive for five years or more after initial diagnosis.

In **Stage 2** bladder cancer, which is signified by cancer cell growth through connective tissue and into bladder wall muscle, half of men and a third of women survive for at least five years after diagnosis.

The survival rates for **Stages 3 and 4** are, unsurprisingly, lower. Stage 3 rates are 30% for men and around 15% for women. At this point, the cancer has spread from the muscle into fat and also could now be outside the bladder itself, in the prostate, womb or vagina.

The most serious stage of cancer (Stage 4) is where the cancer has reached the patient's abdomen, pelvis and/or lymph nodes. Five-year survival rates here are only 10% for both men and women. At Stage 4, bladder cancer might also have spread to other areas of the body, including the bones, liver or lungs. This is undoubtedly why early detection and treatment are imperative.

Understanding risk factors

A 'risk factor' is anything that can increase your risk of getting a particular illness or disease. Some risk factors relate to changes we can make ourselves (e.g. stopping smoking, changing to a healthy diet, exercising more), whilst others are predetermined, such as a family history of a condition, gender or age. However, having one or more risk factors doesn't mean you're definitely going to get an illness. This is why

---

doctors and scientists discuss risk factors instead of causes per se, as everyone will have their unique set of risk factors, and for many conditions, causes are multiple. One person could have only a single risk factor and become unwell, while another might have numerous and stay well. In addition, not all of them are equal in terms of how much they are likely to increase the chances of someone developing an illness. In other words, the 'calculation' for working out our risk is very complicated! Hence, there are some unknowns, which is why it's important to make positive lifestyle changes. These can be understood as 'protective factors', such as eating enough fruit and vegetables each day. In most conditions, eating well, exercising, not smoking or drinking too much alcohol and reducing stress can be viewed as protective factors.

What are the risk factors for bladder cancer?

We have divided this section into risks that we can change or modify and those which we can't. If you have some risk factors that cannot be modified and you're worried about developing bladder cancer, it would be worth seeing your doctor and discussing this with her. But do bear in mind that bladder cancer is uncommon – even if someone in your family has had it, this doesn't mean you will get it.

Modifiable risk factors for bladder cancer

Smoking

By far the biggest risk factor for bladder cancer is cigarette smoking, accounting for half of all cases in developed countries.[82] The good thing about this is that it is possible to stop – in other words, smoking is a modifiable risk factor. There is a great deal of support to help you stop smoking, from smoking-cessation clinics to nicotine-replacement patches and gums. Your doctor will be able to point you in the direction of local services and support you while you're quitting. Also, see the useful addresses section on page 202 for additional sources of information.

People who smoke cigarettes are four times more likely to develop bladder cancer than non-smokers.[83] Pipe and cigar smoking are also problematic. If you started smoking when young, have smoked for many years and smoke heavily, you have the highest risk. This is because the more someone smokes, the more chemicals called arylamines enter the bloodstream and eventually pass through to the urine. Urine of course sits within the bladder so the chemicals touch the lining of the bladder wall.

Chemicals (at work, in hair dye and water disinfectant)

Exposure to chemicals at work is understood to account for 20% of all bladder cancers.[84] This is the second most influential risk factor for bladder cancer after smoking. There are certain groups of chemicals used in the workplace that are now known to increase the risk of bladder cancer – these are arylamines and polycyclic aromatic hydrocarbons (PAHs). Many of these types of chemicals are now illegal, but seeing as bladder cancer can take many years to develop, you may want to discuss this with your doctor if you've worked in rubber or plastics manufacturing, smelting or work that includes combustion, or have handled carbon or crude oil.

Some other, more common jobs/professions may put you in contact with chemicals that can contribute to the development of bladder cancer. These are:
- miners
- mechanics
- painter and decorators
- bus and taxi drivers
- railway workers
- metal casters, machine setters and operators
- people who work with leather
- blacksmiths
- hairdressers.

It may seem strange that hairdressers are included on this list, but it's because they work with chemicals regularly in the form of hair dye. Some of the substances in hair dyes that were found to be carcinogenic have since been banned and many hairdressers take precautions by not touching dye directly. However, research has shown that hairdressers working with hair dyes can have an increased risk of being diagnosed with bladder cancer.[85] If you do any sort of job where you're regularly in contact with chemicals and are worried about cancer, arrange to discuss this with your doctor.

In terms of simply having your hair dyed, the research we have to date is mixed. Some studies show a heightened risk,[85] whilst others show no increase in bladder cancer at all.[86] Therefore, if you have no other risk factors, then using hair dye is probably nothing to worry about. However, if you want to be cautious, there are many natural dyes on the market that use plant ingredients and henna as a colourant instead of chemicals.

The other types of chemicals that researchers have been concerned about are trihalomethanes (THMs), which are a by-product of chlorine. Chlorine plays an important part in drinking water and swimming pools because it stops harmful bacteria populating the water. Like the studies on using hair dye, the results have been inconsistent. However, as we need to disinfect our water, overall the benefits of using chlorine outweigh the risks and much of it can be filtered out with a water filter if you prefer.

Food and drink

Unsurprisingly, a diet high in fruit and vegetables can act as a protective factor against bladder cancer.[82] The current advice is to eat 10 portions of fruit and vegetables each day, which can seem quite difficult. Try to include fruit and veg into every meal and use short-cuts such as frozen veggies to up the intake. Cruciferous vegetables, such as broccoli, Brussels sprouts, cabbage, cauliflower and kale, appear to be particularly beneficial in terms of bladder cancer.

Drinking green and black tea may also help reduce the risk of bladder cancer. Choosing cultured skimmed milk and other fermented dairy products has shown to be protective against bladder cancer whereas full-fat milk has been shown to contribute to risk (see Chapter 10, page 116 for a list of fermented and probiotic foods). Cutting down on processed meat, such as ham and sausages, can also benefit not only bladder health but all-round health too. Alcohol use doesn't appear to be associated with bladder cancer.

In terms of vitamins and minerals, people who have high levels of vitamin A, vitamin D and selenium have a lower risk of developing bladder cancer, but the benefits of using supplements to increase the amounts of these vitamins and mineral are still in question. Vitamin A is high in orange vegetables, such as carrots, and selenium is particularly plentiful in Brazil nuts and sea food. Soak up some sunshine for vitamin D (see page 166).

Body weight

Being overweight doesn't seem to increase the risk of being diagnosed with bladder cancer on its own. However, recent research from the USA found that in people who smoke, being overweight did increase the risk of bladder cancer coming back.[87] As the recurrence rates of bladder cancer can be as high as 40%,[88] this is especially important in this kind of cancer. Furthermore, being obese (defined as someone with a BMI (body mass index) of 30 or more) is related to a higher risk of getting bladder cancer.[89] Therefore, along with giving up smoking, tackling weight gain is a good way to prevent bladder cancer and its recurrence.

Exercise

Being physically active is another protective factor against bladder cancer. Exercising can reduce the risk of bladder cancer by up to 34%.[90] Physical activity can also improve overall quality of life in people that have recovered from bladder cancer.[91]

Unmodifiable risk factors for bladder cancer

Family history

If someone in your family has had bladder cancer it can be very frightening and cause worries about your own health and likelihood of developing the same condition. However, the type of bladder cancer which is caused by a genetic mutation is extremely rare. Also, family history is a risk factor – not a *fait accompli*. It may seem that certain cancers run in families but this is probably because members of the same family behave in similar ways, such as smoking, eating an unhealthy diet, alcohol use, etcetera.

If you have a close relative (first-degree – that is, parent, child, siblings) who has had bladder cancer you are at a higher risk of developing the condition,[92] but if your relative was older than 45 when s/he received a diagnosis, then it is more probable that a combination of environmental and behavioural risk factors led to the disease than a faulty gene.

Other cancer treatments

Unfortunately, the treatments for other types of cancer, such as cervical, prostate, fallopian tube, testicular and womb cancers, can increase the risk of developing bladder cancer. This is usually due to radiotherapy being targeted around the pelvic area, which of course is near the bladder. Some other types of cancers, such as lung, kidney and head/neck cancer, also seem to make it more likely that bladder cancer will occur. However, it's not clear if this is because of radiotherapy and chemotherapy treatment (in the latter a drug called cyclophosphamide appears to be the culprit), or whether all these different kinds of cancer share other risk factors. We of course know that smoking is a risk factor for many cancers so this may well be the case, or alternatively both assertions may be true. Regardless, if you are being treated for any type of cancer ask your doctor to explain your individual set of risk factors as everyone is different.

Other medical conditions

If you have diabetes, you are more likely to get bladder cancer than someone who doesn't have this condition.[93] The stage of diabetes and its treatment account for this increased risk. In type 2 diabetes, a medication called pioglitazone is used to lower levels of sugar in the blood and also increases the action of insulin in cells. However, this drug can have some serious side effects, including weight gain and in some cases congestive heart failure.[94] The longer pioglitazone is used, the greater the risk of bladder cancer. However, other medicines in the thiazolidinedione category, to which pioglitazone belongs, do not appear to be a risk factor for bladder cancer.

People with conditions that require a long-term urinary catheter, such as spinal cord injury, have a higher risk of bladder cancer,[95] as do those who have had a kidney transplant.[96] The latter may again be due to medications – in this case immunosuppressive drugs known as thiopurines.[97] These types of drugs are also used for inflammatory bowel diseases, such as Crohn's disease, which may account for the higher rates of bladder cancer in people with Crohn's disease.[98]

Infections

People who have had numerous bladder infections often worry that they will get bladder cancer. Early research studies seemed to support this concern, but more up-to-date research is now saying that there's no greater likelihood of someone who has suffered from recurrent infections getting bladder cancer.[99] Only a parasitic infection from areas of Africa, the Middle East, Asia and South America has been shown to be related to bladder cancer – this is the condition schistosomiasis (also called 'snail fever' or 'bilharzia') which is caused by the *Schistosoma haematobium* parasitic flatworm and does seem to increase the risk of bladder cancer.

In men, the sexually transmitted infection gonorrhoea can double the risk of developing bladder cancer.[100] In men who smoke this increase appears even higher. Therefore, safe sex practices can be viewed as a proactive factor against bladder cancer for men.

Does the experience of bladder cancer differ from other cancers?

Everyone's experience of cancer is different. Not only do our bodies differ, but the way we cope, the support we have and our outlook can be vastly different from others', even those close to us. When researchers talked to people who had been diagnosed with different types of cancer, there didn't seem to be fundamental variations in how they made sense of their illness experience.[101] Some people felt that cancer was simply part of life's journey while others took something positive from the experience. Importantly, those who did seem to be able to find a silver lining had better overall quality of life. And we know that enhanced quality of life can help many aspects of life, including relationships, psychological wellbeing and everyday functioning. In this way our minds, or rather the way we perceive events (even very frightening and disruptive experiences like cancer), can make a difference.

Summary and conclusion

In this chapter, we have looked in detail at the risk factors associated with bladder cancer. Many of these are modifiable, which is advantageous as we can make positive and real steps to protect our health. However, this doesn't mean that if someone has lived an ultra-healthy life s/he definitely won't develop bladder cancer. Regrettably, some people will get cancer even if they are very low risk, which is one reason why cancer is so frightening. However, bladder cancer is not common and even if someone in your family has had this type of cancer, there is no reason to think you will, especially if you tackle the risk factors that can be modified. If you're worried about bladder cancer or any other type of cancer, the best thing to do is talk to your doctor, who can explain your individual risk factors. Most likely she will put your mind at rest.

In the next chapter, we look at how bladder problems are diagnosed.

Chapter 8

Medical investigations

Some bladder conditions can be difficult to diagnose because they mimic other illnesses. For instance, interstitial cystitis (IC – see page 64) can take on average three to seven years to be diagnosed by a specialist.[102] This is why it's very important to provide your doctor with accurate information about your symptoms and triggers. However, even with the most precise symptom diary and explanation of sensations, some conditions are challenging to identify correctly.

What should you expect when you go to see your doctor?

Your doctor will need to know the characteristics of your bladder symptoms:

- **Pain** – Is this a numb ache? Is there a burning, stinging or sharp pain? Or is the pain more like an uncomfortable sensation? Where exactly is the pain? Your pelvic region or back, for example?
- **Urgency** – We all feel the need to go/race to the toilet now and then, but if you feel ready to burst most of the time and it doesn't seem to be related to the amount you've had to drink, then this should be discussed with your doctor.

- **Nocturia** – Do you have to get up to go to the toilet at night? How often?
- **Frequency** – How often do *all* the symptoms occur?

It's also useful to let your doctor know if anything relieves these symptoms, including when you go to the toilet. If after you've emptied your bladder the symptoms return quickly, tell the GP or specialist this also.

Bladder diary

A bladder diary can be used to provide detailed information about your symptoms to your doctor and can also be used when trying bladder retraining to track progress (see Chapter 9). Your doctor will tell you for how long he wants you to fill out the diary, but it's usually a minimum of three days and up to two weeks. You could start doing this while waiting to see your doctor.

Start by noting down what and how much you drink, either in millilitres or in cups/glasses. This should be entered into the column labelled 'In' in the bladder diary (see Figure 6). You'll also need to record how much urine you pass – you'll need a measuring jug for this. Add the amount of urine into the 'Out' column of the diary.

The next column of the diary is called 'Wet' and refers to leakage. If there have been any leaks simply place a tick next to the time this occurred.

Finally, sensations of urgency should be noted in the final column of the diary. Use the following categories:

A. I felt no need to empty my bladder but did so for other reasons, e.g. because I felt I should wee before going out for the day.

B. I could postpone voiding (emptying my bladder) as

long as necessary without fear of wetting myself.

C. I could postpone voiding for a short while, without fear of wetting myself.

D. I could not postpone voiding, but had to rush to the toilet in order not to wet myself.

E. I leaked before arriving at the toilet.[103]

Day 1				
Time	In	Out	Wet	Urgency
07.00		250 ml	✓	E
08.00	Coffee, 1 cup			
09.00				
10.00		200 ml		C
11.00	Orange juice, 2 cups			
Etc.				

Figure 6: An example of a bladder diary

Cystoscopy

If your urologist needs to see directly inside your bladder, s/he may want to perform a procedure called a 'cystoscopy'. This uses a thin, fibreoptic tube called a 'cystoscope' that is inserted into the urethra (the tube-like structure that carries urine out of the body, see Chapter 2, page 24), and which contains a camera. There are two types of cystoscope – a flexible and a rigid version. The rigid cystoscope has the additional functions of taking biopsies and treating conditions such as bladder stones (by removal). The two kinds of cystoscope also differ in the anaesthetic required when they are used:

- **a rigid cystoscopy** is performed under general anaesthetic or an epidural (spinal anaesthetic);

- **a flexible cystoscopy** uses local anaesthetic, such as a gel substance or spray to limit urethral discomfort.

> Cystoscopy is what I like to call a 'periscope for the bladder'. Well not really, but it reminds me of it; it is a type of endoscope that is inserted into your urethra and bladder, so the doctor can see the inside of the organ and search for any abnormalities.
>
> *Martine*

What conditions can be identified with a cystoscopy?

Cystoscopy may be used to diagnose (or keep track of) a number of conditions. These include:

- interstitial cystitis (IC – see page 64)
- polyps in the bladder (these are non-cancerous growths)
- bladder stones
- a blockage or narrowing of the urethra (the tube that carries urine from the bladder out of the body, see page 19)
- issues with the ureters (the tubes that carry urine from the kidneys to the bladder, see page 19)
- in men, an enlarged prostate gland
- bladder cancer.

How do I prepare for a cystoscopy?

Both the ridged and flexible cystoscopy can be carried out on an out-patient basis and usually patients can go home on the same day. If you have a rigid cystoscopy, you may be asked not to eat or drink before the procedure – usually you'll need to have a completely empty stomach so this means not eating or drinking for several hours, or at all on the day of your appointment, depending on the time the cystoscopy is scheduled. However, if you're asked to undergo a flexible cystoscopy then you should be able to eat and drink as normal on the day.

While most prescription medications will not interfere with the investigation, if you take medicines such as aspirin, ibuprofen or warfarin you should discuss this with your doctor. You may be asked to refrain from taking these medications as they can lead to heavy bleeding during the cystoscopy.

What will happen on the day of the cystoscopy?

Before the cystoscopy, the doctor performing the procedure will explain what will happen. If you have any questions you'll be offered the chance to ask and/or tell the doctor about any concerns you have. If you do have concerns, it can be useful to write these down beforehand as sometimes people feel a little overwhelmed in medical environments. There are no silly questions and the doctor will be happy to chat through any worries you have.

Then, you'll be asked to sign a consent form which states that you've understood the nature of the investigation and any risks associated with it. Give yourself time to read this document – you don't need to rush through it. Again, if anything is unclear do voice your concerns.

To prepare for the cystoscopy you'll be asked to change into a medical gown. So that the procedure can continue unimpeded you might also be asked to provide a urine sample which will be tested for any signs of an infection. The cystoscopy may be rescheduled if you have an infection in the urinary tract.

What will the doctor do during the cystoscopy?

Once the anaesthetic has taken effect, the cystoscope will be well lubricated and inserted into your urethra. The instrument will then be manoeuvred into your bladder. Once in place, sterile water is injected into the bladder to open it up like a balloon. This allows the doctor a clear view of the inside of your bladder.

The amount of time the cystoscope will be placed in the bladder depends on the reason for the procedure; if it is a straightforward investigation, this should only be a matter of minutes (two to 10). However, if the doctor wants to use additional techniques, such as taking an X-ray, the entire cystoscopy will take longer. As this is an invasive procedure you will most likely need to have the entire day off to get to the hospital, have the cystoscopy and then rest at home.

What additional procedures might be carried out during a cystoscopy?

Because a cystoscopy can be used for a number of problems relating to the urinary system, your doctor might also perform one of the following procedures in addition to viewing the inside of your bladder:

- take out a bladder or ureter stone
- take a sample of urine from each ureter to check for infection or a tumour
- take a biopsy (a sample of tissue) from the bladder which can then be examined in a laboratory to test for cancer
- if one of the ureters is narrowed, a small tube called a stent may be placed in it, or if there is a stent already in position, this can be removed via a cystoscopy – this can help with the flow of urine from the kidney to the bladder
- if there is evidence that urine is flowing back up the ureters, medications might be injected to treat this problem
- specialist dye might be used to show blockages or kidney stones on an X-ray.

Is a cystoscopy painful?

In general, the procedure isn't painful, but there can be a burning sensation when the cystoscope is inserted and removed if local anaesthetic has been used. If the cystoscopy has required general anaesthetic or an epidural you won't experience this sensation but you will need to remain under observation of the healthcare staff until you can walk (in the case of general anaesthetic), and until feeling and movement below your chest return in the case of an epidural (both around an hour). For both types of cystoscopy, you'll be able to eat and drink immediately afterwards.

When the doctor fills your bladder with sterile water it may give you a cool sensation or you may feel as though your bladder is uncomfortably full. Relaxation techniques (Chapter 15, page 171) can help to calm the body and take your mind off these sensations.

Will there be any after effects following a cystoscopy?

Overall, most people say that this procedure isn't as bad as they thought it would be. The idea of it is of course unpleasant but it shouldn't be painful and can bring about a diagnosis which, in turn, may lead to long-term relief from your bladder symptoms. You may feel a little nauseous and tired after the general anaesthetic and there can be discomfort and slight backache after the epidural, but this shouldn't last long. Also, because the doctor pumps sterile water into the bladder during the cystoscopy, you may feel the urge to use the toilet once the procedure has finished. In the short term (up to a few days), there may be some blood passed after the cystoscopy but this is normal and not a sign that something is wrong.

What are the risks associated with a cystoscopy?

Cystoscopies are very safe medical procedures. There are always risks associated with a general anaesthetic so if you are worried about these discuss them with your doctor – but know that serious risks and complications are rare.

The most frequent risk associated with a cystoscopy is a brief swelling of the urethra. Swelling may cause urinary retention and if this happens your doctor may want to insert a catheter to drain urine until the swelling dissipates. However, this is rare in women, but men who have already had problems with emptying their bladders may be at increased risk.

Mild UTIs/cystitis can occur after a cystoscopy and will be treated with antibiotics, if appropriate (see Box on page 63). In *extremely* rare cases a puncture to the bladder or urethra may occur which will need surgical intervention. If you are worried about any of these issues and you are in the UK you can compare NHS hospitals in your area (www.nhs.uk/service-search/Hospital/LocationSearch/7/Procedures), or request this type of information from individual service providers.

Although adverse effects are unlikely following a cystoscopy, if you have any of the following symptoms you should contact your GP or consultant:

- There is heavy bleeding or you notice blood clots after emptying your bladder several times (although a pink hue to the urine even for several days after the procedure is normal, particularly if a biopsy was taken).
- Signs of a kidney infection, including a fever or chills; pain in your abdomen or back.
- Urinating has been impossible for eight hours after the cystoscopy.
- You have the symptoms of cystitis (Chapter 6, page 64).

Urodynamic testing

While a cystoscopy is a structural test that looks for any growths, lesions or inflammation in the bladder, there are tests that look at how the bladder functions. This group of tests is known as urodynamic tests (or testing) and aims to discover what's going on in the bladder when it fills with urine and when it's emptied.

To achieve this, the tests must recreate the symptoms a patient experiences – although this can be unpleasant it's sometimes the only way for healthcare professionals to find out what's up with your bladder. Urodynamic tests usually check:

- how much urine passes through the bladder over time (flow rate)
- pressure in the bladder and abdomen (filling cystometry).

These tests are usually done in the same session and analysed in conjunction with a bladder diary (see page 85).

What conditions can be identified with urodynamic testing?

As this type of investigation looks at the function of your bladder, conditions that are caused by differences in the way the bladder works can be evaluated by urodynamic testing, such as:

- in men, an enlarged prostate gland (benign prostatic hyperplasia)
- unstable detrusor muscle
- stress incontinence
- urge incontinence
- mixed stress and urge incontinence.

Investigations such as urodynamic testing can also provide important information about the severity of a bladder problem, particularly if you don't fit the usual criteria for a condition:

> The hospital I went to sort of poo-pooed me – they said, 'You're too young to have a bladder condition as severe as that.' Then they gave me a test where I sat on a toilet and I remember after the test the doctor said to me, 'I can't believe that it is quite so severe,' and he apologised that he had thought I was, well, sort of making it up really.
>
> *Denny*

How do I prepare for urodynamic testing?

If you take medication for your bladder symptoms, your doctor may ask you to stop taking this for five days before your testing session. (Examples of bladder medications can be reviewed in Chapter 12.) It is important that you know for certain if you do need to stop taking these medicines as in some cases your doctor will need to perform the urodynamic tests when you are taking the tablets as prescribed. Therefore, if you are unsure about whether you need to stop taking them, do contact the clinic or hospital where the testing will take place, or your GP.

You will need to complete the bladder diary for at least three days before the investigations. In most cases these do not need to be three consecutive days.

Constipation may interfere with the urodynamic testing. If you do experience constipation in the days before your appointment, see page 128 on how to deal with this problem and discuss these treatments with your doctor.

What will happen on the day of the urodynamic testing?

As mentioned above, urodynamic investigation consists of a flow rate test and a filling cystometry test.

Flow rate

You will generally be asked to attend the appointment with a comfortably full bladder. Of course, your symptoms may make this impossible and if so, you can drink water when you arrive (you'll simply need to arrive early as it takes time for the bladder to fill). Then, you will need to empty your bladder in a special toilet called a flowmeter that measures the amount and rate urine is expelled – this information is sent directly to a computer that analyses the flow and can evaluate any irregularities. This test can demonstrate if there may be a blockage or if the bladder muscles aren't working correctly.

After your bladder has been emptied you may undergo an ultrasound test to see if there is any urine remaining in your bladder, even if you feel your bladder is empty. This is a painless procedure and requires you to simply lie back while the technician moves a lubricated probe over your skin.

Cystometry

In the filling cystometry part of the investigation, catheters are used to see how the bladder fills up. One catheter is inserted into the urethra and the other into the rectum (back passage). Then, the catheters are connected to a bag of fluid – this fluid is squeezed into the bladder in a controlled way to see how the bladder fills. Next the pressure both on the inside and outside of the bladder is measured. This may sound quite unpleasant, but only a small amount of liquid is inserted into the back passage. The nurse or technician will ask you how you're feeling when the bladder is being filled. This is then compared with the reading on the pressure gauge which will show whether you're accurately sensing what's going on in your bladder when it fills up.

> The test [I had done] was urodynamic testing. Cystometry – a clinical diagnostic procedure used to evaluate bladder function. Specifically, it measures the contractile force of the bladder when voiding. The nurse inserts a small tube (like a catheter tube) inside your urethra, which is painless – you feel only a little burn when the tube is inserted. Your bladder is then filled with liquid to see its capacity. You will be asked if you feel the presence of liquid in your bladder and the doctor will be able to see if your bladder feels the liquid on a cystometrogram. You will be asked to cough in order for him/her to see if you have incontinence/leak. Your bladder gets filled until it reaches full capacity. Then you will be asked to use a special toilet that measures the amount of the liquid you have voided to determine if you have voided completely.
>
> *Martine*

What will the nurse do during the urodynamic testing?

Once your bladder is full, the healthcare practitioner might take an X-ray. You could be asked to cough to see if this affects your bladder – that is, it might demonstrate that you have stress incontinence. Because urodynamic testing is an investigation, rather than any type of operation, the nurse will mainly be asking you questions and making notes. Therefore, in addition to the bladder diary, if you experience any sensations or leaking, do tell the nurse as this is vital information regarding what's up with your bladder.

At the end of the testing you will be asked to urinate with the catheters in place to see how the bladder empties. This will be done into the flowmeter again so the amount of fluid passed can be measured accurately.

Is urodynamic testing painful?

Although an anaesthetic gel is used when the catheters are inserted, you may feel a little stinging sensation at first (but only for a few seconds). When the bladder is filled, this may be uncomfortable, particularly if this discomfort is one of your symptoms.

It's important to remember that even though having to wee in a clinical environment isn't an experience we would want and can feel embarrassing, it is the best way to find out if there is a functional disorder. If there is any leaking during the procedure that too is important for the nurse to document as it gives your urologist vital information that can lead to a diagnosis.

Will there be any after effects following urodynamic testing?

You may have some bleeding when you urinate, but this should pass quickly. If it lasts more than 24 hours, it may be a sign of an infection. To avoid the chance of an infection you may want to:

- Flush your urinary system out for two days after the tests by drinking two and a half litres of water each day (this amounts to about nine to 10 cups).
- Cut down or eliminate caffeine, again for two days after the urodynamic testing. Caffeine can irritate the bladder so opt for herbal teas, diluted juice or squash instead. Some people find that decaffeinated tea and coffee also aggravate their bladder so it might be worth avoiding these too after the testing.
- Completely empty your bladder when going to the toilet by taking your time. You can also stand up for a moment then try again to ensure all the urine has been passed.

If you do think you have cystitis after the testing please see your GP.

What are the risks associated with urodynamic testing?

This type of investigation is very safe. However, if you are pregnant or think you might be, tell your doctor as some patients have an X-ray taken during the urodynamic testing. X-rays pose a risk to an unborn baby due to the radiation – but this risk is very small. However, as with any medical procedure and medication, your doctor should be made aware of a pregnancy.

Summary and conclusion

Bladder conditions can be embarrassing and so the investigations and procedures involved in getting a diagnosis can also cause a sense of shame and embarrassment. However, without this information it can be difficult for your doctor to know exactly what the problem is and, subsequently, which is the correct treatment plan for you. We know that people who have a diagnosis have a better quality of life overall so it's important to have any tests your doctor suggests. If you feel overwhelmed with the thought of these tests, it would be worth speaking to some other people who have had them. Organisations such as the Bladder Health UK can put you in touch with others (see Appendix 1, page 202 for details).

In the next chapter, we explore some behavioural treatments that can help control bladder symptoms.

Chapter 9

Behavioural treatments

Behavioral methods… appear to be at least as effective in terms of reducing incontinence episodes as currently available drug therapy.

Kathryn Burgio, PhD, Director,
UAB Continence Program, Professor of Medicine,
University of Alabama at Birmingham[104]

This chapter sets out behavioural methods which can help you regain control of your bladder. The most usual technique is bladder training, which involves, once you have the urge to wee, deliberately stopping yourself from weeing for a certain amount of time. In order to do this, you will need to have techniques at your command to ensure you can do this. One powerful technique is pelvic floor (Kegel) exercises. Many people have found behavioural techniques very helpful, and in this chapter, we present evidence from studies which have been carried out, to determine whether the methods have been shown to really work.

These are the behavioural treatments which we will be discussing.

- Bladder training: delaying emptying of bladder
- Pelvic muscle training (Kegel exercises)
- Monitoring with bladder diaries

- Urge suppression techniques
- Techniques for use during night time.

Bladder training

Bladder training involves delaying voiding/emptying the bladder. This technique is usually accompanied by keeping a bladder diary where you list the time you felt the urge to wee, how long you could wait before you actually did wee, and the time between subsequent wees.

The idea of bladder training is to try to leave a bit more time before you empty your bladder, once you have felt the urge to do so. It's good to keep a bladder diary for a week or so first, so before you try any bladder training, keep a journal (see page 85). This will enable you to see how much progress you make once you start bladder training.

We'll assume you've already started your journal, but haven't yet started bladder training. There are two main types of bladder training you can do:

1. Delaying emptying your bladder for gradually lengthening periods of time
2. Scheduled bladder trips, where you empty your bladder whether or not it is necessary.

Here are examples of the above methods:

Delayed emptying

Imagine you have just got up, and you empty your bladder at 8.00 am, for instance. Perhaps you have a cup of tea or coffee and find you have an urge to wee at 9.00. Bladder training requires you to try to hold out, say, until 9.05, or 9.07, whichever you can do without being in agony. At first it's hard to do this. Don't of course hold on so much that you fail to reach the toilet when you do need it! So you need to have a realistic goal. Maybe you can only hold on until 9.05. The next time you need a wee, you might hold on for another minute. Note it down in your journal. Many people monitor the amount of urine they empty each time (an old measuring jug is useful here). This is good because it will show (we hope) that at the beginning of training, you needed to wee when your bladder was (say) 100 ml full, but after a few days/weeks, you find you do not need to wee until your bladder is 250 ml full, and perhaps eventually, 300 ml full (more for men). Do drink and eat normally when you're trying this technique. If you feel you need to wee during the intervals, then you can use urge suppression techniques, which are ways of occupying your mind and body so that you can hold on for longer. Such techniques are listed later in this chapter.

Hahn-Ey Lee and colleagues in Seoul in South Korea decided to see whether such training was successful or not.[105] Their sample was 105 patients with overactive bladder (OAB), both men and women. Their bladder training (BT) programme consisted of the participants writing in a bladder diary, not going to wee as soon as they felt the urge to go, distracting themselves from thinking about weeing, and performing the Kegel exercises five to six times. The participants also filled in various bladder and health questionnaires. The researchers say that after the first BT programme, results showed improvements in frequency, urgency and getting up in the night. Further improvements were shown after the second BT programme, and diaries showed that there were significant changes in the amounts the participants' bladders held before needing to void, between the first and the second BT programmes. The authors stated that almost all of the people in the study said that BT had improved their symptoms.

Scheduled bladder trips (timed voiding)

This is similar to the above, except that you decide on regular times when you will empty your bladder, so perhaps on the first day, you decide you will wee every hour. This means that at 8.00 am and every hour until bed, you empty your bladder, even though you might not need to go. The time elapsed is then lengthened for the following days – for example, on the next few days you might go every one hour 15 minutes, and the following days, every one and a half hours.

Needless to say, you should keep a journal so that you can monitor your progress.

You will need to decide whether in your particular situation, scheduled bladder trips or delaying bladder emptying gives the better results. Many people have found their problems improved with these techniques.

The final goal of bladder training is to need to empty your bladder only once every three hours or so. Of course, there are always going to be times when you need to go much more often – usually connected with food / drinks / infections.

Just thinking about not going to the toilet isn't very helpful in bladder training, so you need to use the right techniques to help you hold on.

Pelvic floor muscle training (Kegel exercises)

> I get really excited about undercarriages because physio is such effective treatment. There is oodles of gold-standard research showing that physiotherapy helps vaginal prolapse, bladder and bowel incontinence and sexual dysfunctions.
>
> Elaine Miller[106]

Pelvic floor exercises are particularly important for pregnant women as being pregnant and giving birth can damage the muscles which control the flow of urine (Chapter 2). A large-scale review showed that using these exercises can prevent urinary incontinence up to six months after delivery in women having their first baby, and may be especially useful to women who have a higher risk of incontinence, such as those having a large baby or those who are anticipating a forceps delivery.[107]

Furthermore, both men and women with bladder dysfunction can be helped by carrying out the exercises. Kegels are easy to do. However, you need to find the right muscles. One of the easiest ways to locate your muscles is when you wee. Here's how:

- Squeeze the muscles you use to stop your urine; halfway through weeing, stop or slow down the flow.
- Don't hold your breath or tense your other muscles.
- If you can slow or stop the flow, then these are the muscles you use for the pelvic floor exercises.

To begin the exercises:
- First, lie down on your back on a flat surface, such as the floor or bed.
- Squeeze the muscles for 2 seconds, then relax for 2 seconds.
- After 2 seconds, add 1 second each week until you are able to squeeze for 10 seconds.
- Repeat the exercise 10 to 15 times a session. Do at least three sessions a day.

After a while you should try to do the exercises standing up, sitting up, in the car – wherever and as often as you can (see the Hold Tight campaign below).

There is evidence that this is very helpful to people with urinary incontinence. A recent study in Turkey studied 72 women. Thirty-eight of the women had stress incontinence and 34 were a mixed urinary incontinence group. They used Kegel exercises which consisted of 10 sets of contractions a day. Each set included 10 repetitions for at least eight weeks. After the study, 68% of the women with stress incontinence and 41% of the women in the mixed group had significant improvements.[108] The authors stated that this was an effective treatment, especially as the exercises can be done at home or work without any supervision.

But if you'd like to get some help with pelvic floor exercises, an exercise programme created in Finland is being rolled out in the UK. This is what Nora Thoden from Bailamama says about the approach:

The Bailamama health exercise concept was developed in Finland in 2011 by a midwife and a physiotherapist, together with other health and fitness professionals. The objective of Bailamama is to motivate all women to regularly train the pelvic floor muscles in effective and fun ways. It all started from a lack of efficient, effective and fun exercise classes for new mothers with babies that recognised the fact that the recovery from the pregnancy should start from the pelvic floor muscles. The Bailamama exercise classes became very popular and liked by the new mothers and soon new Bailamama classes were introduced. Today, there are live Bailamama group exercise classes, virtual classes as well as home training programmes for three target groups spanning over the different life stages of women: for pregnant women, for new mothers with their babies, and for all health-conscious women regardless of age or fitness level. The overarching concept of Bailamama is to include pelvic floor training in programmes that incorporate music, enjoyable exercises, achievable goals and, in the end, give women a feeling of success and achievement.

In May 2016, Bailamama partnered with the Federation of the Finnish Midwives and the Finnish Society of Obstetrics and Gynaecology and a couple of other research organisations to promote the importance of pelvic floor training in the prevention of urinary incontinence, a very common problem affecting women of different ages. Bailamama and its partners together launched a nationwide 'Hold Tight' campaign that encouraged women to take up a challenge to train pelvic floor muscles whenever at a red traffic light, whether driving a car or walking. This method of conditioning the brain to pelvic floor training whenever at a red light has been long used by Dr. Pirkko Brusila, a Finnish gynaecologist and sexual therapist, to teach women to regularly train the pelvic floor muscles. Thousands of women in Finland have taken up the 'Hold Tight' challenge so far.

If a class isn't for you, there is an app called Squeezy which was designed by chartered physiotherapists specialising in both women's and men's pelvic health and developed by the NHS (www.squeezyapp.co.uk/). The app includes audio and visual guidance to help you do pelvic floor exercises that are tailored to your specific needs. Alternatively, you can access free exercise guides and much more information about the pelvic floor from The Continence Foundation of Australia, a government-funded website that is regularly updated with the most up-to-date evidence and techniques (www.pelvicfloorfirst.org.au).

Urge suppression techniques

Don't think about an elephant.

What picture just came into your mind? An elephant of course. Herein lies the problem – when we try to stop thinking about something, it invariably pops into our heads.

When you first train your bladder, it can be very hard to hold on. The aim of these techniques is to distract your mind from thinking about your bladder. Try the following techniques and choose the ones which make the most difference to you.

- Sit down on a hard surface

- Cross your legs
- Tighten your pelvic floor muscles
- Count backwards
- Meditate; breathe deeply
- Curl your toes
- Distract yourself by whatever methods you can so you don't think of the bathroom/toilet
- Make a shopping list
- Imagine what you will buy for someone's birthday etc.

Watching TV or reading a book are not usually good ways to distract ourselves as they are rather passive activities. As well as the above examples of distraction methods, you can try what are known as 'grounding techniques'. These are activities that use more mental effort, and in this way are more distracting than watching a programme as you need to concentrate. If you play a musical instrument this is a type of grounding technique. Challenging puzzles or crosswords can also occupy your mind so that you shouldn't focus on the need to wee as much. Even something like pattern needlework, cooking or gardening can be a useful means of distraction. If you're out and about, listing every ice cream flavour, national capital cities or political leaders can prove engrossing enough to shift attention.

When it's okay for you to go to the bathroom/toilet, don't rush; go at a normal pace.

Night time

It's not unusual for people to often have to get up in the night to wee. Many people get up once in the night, sometimes twice. But obviously having to get up regularly in the night, sometimes multiple times, is unusual. OIder people in particular (those over 70) might need to get up twice a night. It seems that after the menopause, oestrogen deficiency can cause changes in the lower urinary tract which can lead to the symptoms of overactive bladder. Although postmenopausal women will still have a certain amount of oestrogen, older people eventually stop producing it altogether.

To limit the number of times you need to go to the toilet in the night, empty your bladder completely before you decide to go to sleep. If you wake up needing to wee, stay in bed, try to go to sleep, count backwards, or meditate. This is bladder training for the night! Hopefully, you will get back to sleep, although you might wake up again feeling as if you need to wee. Again, try to stay in bed and get back to sleep. Of course this might lead to an increased number of toilet dreams! If you feel that you really *must* get up, wait as long as possible before you do. It is difficult to stay in bed when your bladder is telling you to get up, but this, with other techniques such as fluid restriction before bed, and changes to food and drinks (see Chapter 10), will help in getting your bladder under control.

What you shouldn't do

The worst thing you can do is what many of us have done – gone to the toilet 'just in case'. This is generally when you are out and about, when you see a toilet and think, 'If I don't go now, there might not be another opportunity for a while.' And then when the next toilet opportunity presents itself, you empty your bladder again, even though it wasn't necessary.

When someone first gets bladder dysfunction, they tend not to know about this, and when they are at home, they just use the toilet whenever they want, so as soon as the urge comes, they empty their bladder, even if their bladder has hardly anything in it. You can see that this trains the bladder to void when it is hardly full at all. But we've all done it! At least, we – the authors – have. Having said that, there are times when you have to break the just-in-case rule. If you're going out to some sort of performance, such as a lengthy opera, then it makes sense to go to the toilet shortly before the performance. Otherwise, worrying about having to get up and go to the toilet mid-performance is just too stressful. But when you're at home, or out and about in town where there are plenty of toilets in pubs, shops and cafés, you really don't need to worry too much.

Summary and conclusion

We hope we've given you enough information for you to start trying out some or all of the techniques above. Behavioural treatments are often the first option your doctor will suggest you try, as they are effective and don't have the side effects that medications may have. You can of course try these before you consult your GP, along with the suggestions in the next chapter about food and drink. However, don't forget to log everything in your bladder journal so you can see what's helping.

Chapter 10

Food and drink

The ICA Complementary and Alternative Medicine (CAM)
survey of 2000 IC sufferers was carried out in 2009. 80% of
sufferers, and especially newly diagnosed patients, said that
making changes to their diet helped to control their symptoms.
Whilst dietary changes may not be a cure for IC [interstitial
cystitis], identifying and avoiding foods that trigger flares will
help to keep the symptoms under control.

Bladder Health UK

There is often confusion about what types of food and drink
exacerbate bladder problems – for instance, cranberry juice
is commonly cited as a remedy for cystitis but the research
evidence does not support this; furthermore, cranberry products
can worsen some bladder conditions, such as chronic bladder
inflammation. In this chapter, we discuss the foods and drinks
you can consume which can improve your gut microbiota
(see Chapter 4), and whether pre- and probiotics can improve
your bladder health. We talk about foods which are commonly
thought to help your bladder, and those foods which have
been said to irritate it. We discuss whether swapping to an
alkaline diet may help, and also how to carry out an exclusion/
elimination diet.

What may cause problems

Many people without bladder problems have found that drinking coffee has a diuretic and laxative effect. This is not necessarily problematic for them. However, for people with bladder problems, these effects may be amplified, and the urgency to get to a toilet, especially accompanied by increased frequency, can be highly inconvenient and irritating.

Many people with bladder dysfunction find that some drinks, such as coffee, alcohol and citrus juices, make their symptoms worse, and that spicy foods also affect them. In Bladder Health UK's literature, people are advised to steer clear of a wide variety of foods. Their booklet on the *Bladder-Friendly Diet*, given to everyone who joins, shows lists of foods which are either well tolerated, or should be avoided by people with bladder dysfunction. The following is a condensed version of the foods which they have found should be avoided.

Foods to avoid

Meat and fish
- Most products which are preserved, fast-food or heavily spiced

Dairy products
- Blue cheese or strong cheese
- Chocolate, lemon and strawberry cheesecakes
- Lemon, lime, orange, chocolate or artificially flavoured, sweetened yoghurts

Vegetables
- Baked beans canned in tomato sauce
- Any vegetables pickled in vinegar
- Red tomatoes, tomato paste, sauce or juice

Fruit
- Kiwi fruit
- Lemon juice
- Pineapple
- Preserved prunes

Spices
- Chilli powder
- Yeast extract
- Paprika

General foodstuffs
- Chocolate
- Spicy foods
- Soy products
- Alcohol
- Dried food
- Tomato-based meals
- Worcester sauce
- Vinegars
- Aspartame, NutraSweet, or sugar-free sweets.*

Drinks to avoid

The following is a condensed version of the drinks Bladder Health UK recommend avoiding:
- Citrus/acidic juice (e.g. orange, cranberry, grapefruit drinks)
- All caffeinated and decaffeinated drinks
- Drinking chocolate
- Champagne, sparkling wines
- Carbonated water.

Footnote: We recommend that instead of artificial sweeteners you use products containing stevia leaf.

In the box in Chapter 6 (page 61) we found that cranberries, taken either as juice or supplements, only helped slightly more than doing nothing at all for a one-off bout of cystitis. Using cranberry products to prevent bladder infections is a common self-help suggestion, so it may seem surprising to see cranberry juice listed as something to avoid here. Cranberry juice is quite acidic (pH value around 2.3-2.5) so it may be that for people who have bladder irritation, such as those with IC, this juice will further aggravate the condition. For people who just get the occasional episode of cystitis, cranberry juice may, indeed, prevent bacteria sticking to the bladder wall. Overall though, the scientific evidence for cranberry products for long-term bladder issues is just not there. Hence, if you have a chronic bladder condition, the advice is to avoid this type of fruit juice.

Individual differences

Although most of us find that avoiding certain foods and drinks helps our bladder dysfunction, scientific studies often find that there is no association between foods and drinks and bladder problems. One news item in Australia mentioned a study in which people drank decaffeinated coffee or no caffeine – and there was no difference in any of the bladder measures taken.[109] It seems to be just a case of trying what works best for you, personally. Strangely enough, one study found that beer might have a protective effect in the development of overactive bladder (OAB)![110]

We wondered why there was such a discrepancy between what people were telling us about the foods and drinks which affected their bladders, and the scientific studies which showed there were no effects. Then we remembered a study carried out in 2015 which showed that people found huge differences in the way the same foods affected them. This was a large study in which around 800 people took part, and the researchers gained information on nearly 47,000 meals altogether.[111] What they found was that for some people, a certain food would raise their blood glucose levels, and yet for others, it wouldn't. They gave an example of bread, where some people had high responses, and some experienced no change, and that was the case for any food.

Why should this be? Well, it seems that the differences are due to the differences in our gut microbiota. As we explained in Chapter 4, all of us have different amounts of 'good bacteria' in our guts. We have trillions of these micro-organisms (across between 500 and 1000 species), which have evolved to live with us in our bodies. These micro-organisms are intimately involved in the immune system and are therefore very important to us. Collectively they make up our 'microbiota' and if this gets out of balance (for example, as a result of taking certain antibiotics) then this can lead to increased immune activity. In IBS, this can lead to low-grade inflammation. It is entirely possible that this could happen for UTIs/cystitis also.

This is what experts Cryan & Dinan said:

> It has recently become evident that microbiota, especially microbiota within the gut, can greatly influence all aspects of physiology, including gut-brain communication, brain function and even behaviour. Indeed, the initiation of largescale metagenomic projects, such as the Human Microbiome Project, has allowed the role of the microbiota in health and disease to take centre stage.'[112]

Unfortunately, the microbiota can be adversely affected by various substances, including antibiotics, laxatives, other medications, antiperspirants and artificial sweeteners, as we mentioned before. Disturbances in the gut microbiota have been linked with obesity, depression, diabetes and diseases such as inflammatory bowel disease (IBD) and irritable bowel syndrome

(IBS). However, knowing the importance of the gut microbiota to disease, it's possible that changing the way we eat can actually help IBD, IBS – and bladder problems. Research shows that people with IBS often show abnormal amounts of bad bacteria and/or a restricted number of species. What we need is good diversity of these micro-organisms. We know that pre- and pro-biotics (see page 115) are better at helping with IBS symptoms than placebo. Studies have also shown that certain foodstuffs are good for your microbiota. Luckily for those of us who like chocolate, studies have shown that high-cocoa drinks and high-cocoa chocolate can help: after participants consumed high levels of cocoa, their good bacteria showed a significant increase and their bad bacteria a significant decrease.

In one study, 30 people were given 40 grams of dark chocolate to eat daily for up to 14 days.[113] The researchers took measurements of blood and urine over time and also studied the changes in metabolism due to chocolate consumption. They found that the chocolate improved gut microbial metabolism.

We all have different numbers of various species of microbiota. Some people's microbiota are more diverse than others. The study above[113] shows that people react differently to the same foods. Thus, for some people, drinking chocolate might irritate their bladder; for others, it won't. Researchers normally take a random selection of participants to include in their studies, and it could be that the number of people having a bad reaction to say, tomatoes, will be balanced out by the number of people who don't react badly. Therefore, the study will show little or no effect. If this is true, then people with bladder dysfunction have to take a much more individual approach, using trial and error, or exclusion diets, to find what affects them, although cutting down on the foods and drinks identified by Bladder Health UK is a good starting point.

Exclusion diets

There are various ways of carrying out exclusion diets. There are so many foods, to test each one separately would take a long time, so often exclusion diets take out several foods at once. As Bladder Health UK has given a list of foods and drinks which their members have shown to be well tolerated, or best avoided, perhaps it is a good idea to start with those. Let's say that you want to see if your favourite coffee affects your bladder, and that your favourite foods are tomatoes and blue cheese (all three of which are on Bladder Health UK's 'avoid' list).

The first thing you should do is to keep a food-and-drink symptoms diary. Choose a day to start the diary – at this point you are just recording the effects of foods and drinks.

You'll have a suspicion that coffee is affecting your bladder. Maybe the cheese and tomatoes also? In which case, you need to omit coffee, cheese and tomatoes from your diet for, say, a month. If you find that your bladder is a lot calmer after this time, then you need to find out which of the foods and drinks are responsible for the improvement. This is where you reintroduce the foods/drinks, one at a time. If your symptoms re-appear, you will have evidence that these particular foods/drinks should be eliminated from your daily diet. It's not a good idea to eliminate whole food groups (e.g. all dairy, or all fruits) from your diet. Target the ones that you think are the most likely to be aggravating your bladder. This might be a slow process, but will be very useful in finding out what triggers your bladder problems.

Time of day	Food	Drink	Number of visits to void bladder	Any leakage	Urgency? A = v urgent B = urgent C = not urgent
7–8 am		*Tea*	*1*	*No*	*B*
9–10 am	*Cereal*	*Milk*	*1*	*No*	–
10–1 am		*Coffee*	*3*	*No*	*A*
11–12 am	–		*1*	*No*	*B*
12–1 pm	*Bread, Blue cheese, tomatoes, lettuce*	*Coffee*	*3*	*No*	*A*
1–2 pm					
2–3 pm					
3–4 pm					
5–6 pm					
6–7 pm					
7–8 pm					
8–9 pm					
9–10 pm					
10–11 pm					
11–12 pm					
12–1 am					
1–2 am					

Figure 7: Sample food-and-drink symptom diary

Probiotics and prebiotics

Probiotics are good bacteria, such as *Lactobacilli*, which are found in many foods and which promote a good balance of gut microbiota.

Prebiotics are substances, such as inulin, that are also present in many foods but which enable these good bacteria (probiotics) to thrive. Some foods are rich in both pro- and prebiotics, in which case they are called 'synbiotic'.

Probiotics

Probiotics are live micro-organisms which when ingested improve the balance of your microbiota. They are particularly useful after taking antibiotics, which disturb this balance. They have been shown to be effective for various disorders.[114] Eating live yoghurt will help balance your microbiota, or you can buy supplements in health stores or on websites. However, one scientific review of probiotics concluded that many of the commercial probiotics do not survive in the human gastrointestinal tract (Elmer, 2001).[115] Elmer found one supplement in capsule form did survive in the gastrointestinal tract – Culturelle (produced by CAG functional foods) and produced good effects. In relation to UTIs/cystitis, Elmer said:

> An effective probiotic would have applicability in recurrent and chronic UTI... highly adherent* strains of probiotic microorganisms would seem to be of paramount importance for use in UTIs.

Foods which have probiotic properties include many dairy foods but also other fermented foods:

- milk
- yoghurt
- creme fraiche
- cheeses, especially strong or blue cheeses
- chocolate (high cocoa)
- cocoa
- ice cream
- kefir (a traditional Middle Eastern beverage which can be milk or water based)
- kimchi (a Korean vegetable dish)
- sauerkraut

Footnote: Microbiota that adhere to the urinary tract lining.

- soy foods, soy germ
- pickles
- tempeh (Indonesian dish)
- wheat germ
- turmeric
- green tea
- blueberries
- wheat barley
- malt
- wines
- other fermented foods.

You'll note that quite often foods which help the microbiota are the foods which Bladder Health UK says you should avoid, and vice versa. There's no easy answers here, unfortunately. It's just personal trial and error.

Probiotic supplements

If you decide to take probiotics for a UTI/cystitis, you need to take them daily and preferably over the long term. Studies have shown that probiotics can help with UTIs.[116] One study investigating women with recurrent UTIs found that these occurred in only 15% of women who took probiotics as opposed to 27% who took a placebo.[117]

Prebiotics

Prebiotics nourish the beneficial microorganisms already in the gut. Taking a prebiotic supplement increases the number of bifidobacteria (one type of good bacteria) in the gut. Prebiotics can also stimulate the growth and activity of probiotics. Therefore, it is best to take them together. Foods high in prebiotics are:

- asparagus
- barley

- bananas
- berries
- garlic
- honey
- leeks
- onions
- rye
- seeds
- whole wheat.

Foods and drinks in relation to alkalisation

Our blood and bodily fluids, including urine, can be classified as alkaline, neutral or acidic. This is measured by a pH level. A pH level of 7.00 is neutral. A value above this is alkaline, and below 7.00 is acidic. Human blood should be very slightly alkaline (between 7.35 and 7.45). The pH of urine can vary between 4.5 (acidic) and 8 (alkaline) as it plays its part in keeping blood pH balanced. The types of foodstuffs, drinks, supplements, drugs and chemicals that we consume will push our pH level to either the acidic or alkaline. Bladder Health UK says that a painful bladder can be exacerbated by the urine being too acidic or too alkaline. A study carried out in 2014 lends weight to this as researchers found that having the urine slightly alkaline improved pain and sleep in people with OAB.[118] A study in 2015 looked at 329 patients with OAB and 201 people without.[119] The researchers gave questionnaires and measured 24-hour urinary pH. Some participants underwent a diet programme for four weeks; urine pH values were recorded before the diet and two and four weeks after the diet. They found that 61% of patients with OAB had an acidic urinary pH, and that the presence of acidic urine was related to the condition – that is, those with acidic pH values had worse OAB. They found that alkalisation of urine improved lower urinary tract symptoms

Urine testing

It's very easy to test your urine. You can buy a test kit from Bladder Health UK, or search the internet for the strips of coloured card. You simply take a strip, run the urine over the strip, which will then turn a different colour, allowing you to know how alkaline, or acidic, your urine is. The plan is to alter your diet until you have a neutral, or slightly alkaline reading. It is important not to have a urine pH of more than 8 (this is within the normal range). In order to reach this state, you need to eat lots of alkaline-forming foods (but not eliminate the acid-forming foods).

Which foods are alkaline?

The foods which are alkaline forming are mostly fruit and vegetables. The pH of the food itself is not a good indication of whether it has an alkaline effect. The common example is lemon, which is very acidic, but after being ingested, is alkaline-forming while meat when tested is alkaline but releases acids on being digested. Don't, however, cut out all acid-forming foods. The proportion of alkaline-forming foods should be the majority of what you should eat. Check the pH of your urine to ensure that it is slightly alkaline. Of course, the acidity of urine will vary, just as your temperature varies, so, do your urine test at the same time of day each time, and note whether your bladder problems improve when your urine is slightly alkaline.

A good source of information about the impact on body pH of certain foods can be found at https://trans4mind.com/nutrition/AirWaterLife-FoodImpactOnBody-pH-Chart.pdf.

Water

Drink enough water. There are various guidelines about how much water we should be drinking – for example, one source says nearly two litres a day (see Chapter 11, page 121). Obviously, people differ in the amount they need. When you go to the loo, check the colour of your urine – it should be light yellow. Any darker than that indicates that you are not drinking enough and you might be dehydrated. Sometimes people who have bladder problems deliberately reduce the amount they drink when they are out in order to ensure they won't suddenly need to pee. The key to this is to sip throughout the day rather than drinking, say, 250 ml and then another 250 ml later. Many people choose a time in the evening beyond which they make sure they don't eat or drink in order to reduce the likelihood of needing to get up in the night. The best 'last drink' to have at night is water. Alcohol, tea, coffee, drinking chocolate and especially fruit juices are exactly what you should avoid in order to minimise the chances of nocturia as they can all have a diuretic effect.

Summary and conclusion

This chapter has provided advice about the foods and drinks that you may want to avoid – or include – if you have bladder problems. However, as we have mentioned, different people have different triggers so it would be worth finding out exactly which foods and drinks irritate *your* bladder so that you can exclude or limit them from your diet.

In the next chapter, we look at some further changes you can make to your life to help regain control of bladder function.

Chapter 11

Lifestyle changes

Following on from the previous chapter on diet, in this chapter we explore other changes you can make in your daily life to help control and eliminate bladder symptoms. These suggestions can be used in addition to exercises, such as those that target the pelvic floor (Chapter 9), and medications that your doctor may recommend (Chapter 12). Embarrassing and chronic conditions such as those described in this book can make us feel completely out of control and that our bodies are no longer our own. By making changes to lifestyle, it is possible to regain a sense of control. You may still need medical interventions of course, and altering habits and behaviours is not an easy task, but small changes can help to bring back quality to our lives. Therefore, below we discuss specific (such as fluid intake) and general (such as stress reduction) techniques that can be used to tackle bladder problems.

Fluid intake

How much should I drink a day?

As noted in Chapter 10, drinking water is important for anyone with a bladder condition. Our bodies are mainly water – two-thirds in fact of our physical make-up consist of water so drinking enough is very important. The general guidance from the

European Food Safety Authority (EFSA) recommends consuming two and a half litres of fluid if you're a man and two litres of fluid for women every day, through both food and drink.[120] There has been much debate over whether we should drink only plain water to account for the daily intake or if other drinks can be included in this tally. Some people don't like the taste of water (and in some places water can indeed taste unpleasant) but for our overall health it's important not to replace water with sugary drinks, such as cola and other soft drinks.

As mentioned, water also comes from the food we eat – about 20-30% of our water intake is derived from food sources. As per standard guidance, try to eat a good quantity of fruits and vegetables each day (at least a third of your plate should be this type of food) which will provide your body with additional fluid and also important vitamins and minerals for health and wellbeing.

Does alcohol count as fluid intake?

Although beer, wine, cider, spirits, etc are fluids, our bodies will lose water in the process of trying to eliminate the alcohol. The parched mouth and thumping headache associated with a hangover are the result of our bodies trying to process alcohol – during this process we excrete water to rid ourselves of this toxin, so even if drinking normal strength alcoholic beverages results in an overall fluid gain, it's important to stay within the recommended guidelines of no more than 14 units a week for both men and women. (A standard size glass of wine (175 ml) with an ABV (alcohol by volume) of 12% is 2 units. High strength beer of approximately 5.2% ABV is 3 units, whereas weaker beer of around 3.6% ABV is only 2 units. A small measure of spirits (25 ml) is one unit.)

Should I limit fluid intake if I have bladder problems?

Unless your doctor or specialist has explicitly told you to reduce the amount of fluid you drink, then the answer is usually no. If nocturia (needing to get up and go to the toilet frequently during the night) is one of your symptoms, then you may want to experiment with drinking less in the evenings, but in general, by drinking less, urine becomes more concentrated. Highly concentrated urine can irritate the bladder lining – that is, limiting the amount you drink can exacerbate some bladder problems, for instance interstitial cystitis (IC). Therefore, drinking much earlier in the day, rather than becoming dehydrated, can be a useful strategy, bearing in mind that some beverages, such as citrus juices and carbonated drinks, may make symptoms worse so should be avoided (Chapter 10).

However, many people with bladder problems do stop drinking, particularly if they have to make a long journey. As Martha tells us, this can be counter-productive:

Before I had a diagnosis of bladder inflammation (IC), I thought that if my bladder was empty I would be okay on the train. So I wouldn't drink much, if anything, before work but it didn't really help and I found my symptoms just got worse and worse, until I had to be signed off from work. I felt I had no other choice as I couldn't hold out for an entire class. But it took so long to get a diagnosis that I actually realised myself that my bladder felt less painful when it was – not full – but when I'd been drinking plenty. The problem with that was that if I was in a situation where I was hemmed in (like on a train or in a theatre) I would desperately feel the need to pee. I'd never had panic attacks before but I would say that I had a few before I stopped going out – not because of anxiety on its own, but the thought of wetting myself in public was terrifying.

Martha

Stress and anxiety

Martha's story leads us on to the topic of stress. Dealing with a condition that affects bladder function undoubtedly causes stress. Even if someone doesn't experience incontinence, they may still feel much more anxious and fear having an accident in public. This would be more than embarrassing for most people and mean that those with bladder symptoms stay home, potentially becoming isolated. Isolation itself causes both severe mental health problems, such as depression, and physical health conditions such as heart disease and stroke (to the same extent as smoking). Indeed, depression and stress have been seen to impact quality of life in women with IC.[121] Therefore, dealing with stress effectively can be a vital part of maintaining health and wellbeing in people with or without bladder conditions.

Researchers in California looked at women with 'dry' OAB and compared their anxiety levels with women without a bladder condition. Unsurprisingly, the women with OAB, even though they didn't have accidents, reported higher levels of anxiety.[122] In fact, a large study of 30,000 people demonstrated that 36% of men and 53% of women with bladder problems from the USA, the UK and Sweden met clinical criteria for anxiety.[123]

Why is it important for people with bladder problems to reduce stress?

In Chapter 3, we discussed the relationship between the central and peripheral nervous systems and the bladder. We know the brain and bladder are interconnected and because of this some scientists have proposed that people with anxiety are more likely to develop conditions such as IC. Researchers have used rats that are genetically predisposed to anxiety to see whether these animals felt more bladder pain than rats that were less inclined towards anxious behaviour. When put in a stressful situation (the rats were put in a tank filling with water), the anxious rats exhibited a greater sensitivity to bladder pain. In humans, stressful situations created in a laboratory (difficult mental tasks) showed that those with IC felt more pain and urgency than people without pre-existing bladder symptoms. However, this doesn't mean that those with IC are merely 'sensitive' or 'weak'. Acute and chronic stress can cause some of the mechanisms that we discussed in Chapter 6, such as inflammation, that are found in IC. Hence, the relationship between a condition like IC and stress could be that long-term stress causes physiological changes which make people more prone to develop conditions such as IC, but then these changes, such as the inflammation of the lining of the bladder, cause symptoms, which in turn cause stress (potentially more so in people genetically predisposed to anxiety). Therefore, reducing stress and learning relaxation techniques that help us control anxiety (see Chapter 15) may additionally help us not only feel better emotionally, but also control bladder symptoms.

Smoking

In Chapter 7, we discussed how certain chemicals (arylamines) contained in smoking products enter the bloodstream and pass into the urine, which then sits in the bladder. Whilst this increases the risk of bladder cancer significantly, even in people who don't develop cancer, nicotine can irritate the bladder wall leading to overactive contractions. We have seen in previous chapters in this book that these contractions cause urgency and the need to go to the toilet more often, and potentially urge incontinence (Chapter 5, page 50). People who smoke may develop a 'smoker's cough', a consequence of inflammation in the lungs caused by the toxins in smoking products. Our bodies continually try to rid us of potentially damaging substances –

the smoker's cough is a way in which our lungs endeavour to expel toxins from our respiratory system. In people with bladder problems, particularly those who experience stress incontinence, a hacking cough such as this can cause urine leakage.

What about passive smoking?

If you live in a house with smokers, you may be worried about the effects of passive smoking, in terms of both cancer risk and respiratory problems. While the scientific research doesn't show an association between passive smoking and bladder cancer,[124] you may still want to encourage your loved one to give up smoking as breathing in polluted air is a risk factor for a range of respiratory issues, such as asthma and chronic obstructive pulmonary disease (COPD).[125]

How do I stop smoking?

If you or someone in your family is planning to give up smoking, do take advantage of the support that can be accessed via your doctor and online (see www.nhs.uk/smokefree).

Body weight

As we saw in Chapter 7, obesity appears to be linked to bladder cancer for people who also smoke. Being severely overweight has also been shown to contribute to other bladder conditions, such as OAB. A study of children from five to 12 years old found that in both boys and girls, an overactive bladder was more likely in the children who weighed more.[126] Having a high Body Mass Index (BMI) puts pressure on the bladder and is linked to problems with pelvic floor muscles.[127]

In adults, losing weight can significantly reduce urinary incontinence. Overweight and obese women who lost on average 8% of their body weight (over a healthy period of six months) had almost half as many wetting accidents, compared with before they started the weight-loss programme.[128] The programme included a calorie-controlled diet (1200 to 1500 calories per day, with no more than 30% of the calories coming from fat) and exercise of around 30 minutes a day (brisk walking). The women were also taught some psychological-behavioural skills, such as self-monitoring, stimulus control, and problem-solving. At the end of the programme, the women on this programme said that they found their bladder issues to be less of a problem in their everyday lives.

What's the best way to lose weight?

As with stopping smoking, losing weight can be challenging so take advantage of the support from family and friends to get down to a healthy weight. The above programme was specifically designed and used for a research study so it isn't available to the general public, but there are countless products and programmes on the market for weight loss which help people both shed pounds and, perhaps more importantly, maintain weight loss. Note, however, that many of these studies lack scientific evidence. People using the Weight Watchers programme seem to progress better than those on alternative weight-loss plans, most likely due to a combination of the clear and relatively unrestrictive calorie reduction 'SmartPoints®' diet, weekly weigh-ins and group support. Intermittent fasting diets where you have two very low-calorie days per week (e.g. the 5:2 diet[129]) are also backed-up by research.[130]

Social support is vital in all areas of health so if you'd rather not embark on a paid-for programme, find a friend, or group of friends, to be weight-loss partners – as the encouragement and reassurance will help far more with weight loss than expensive diet products. Finally, if no diets seem to work, look carefully at when you eat and how you're feeling when you eat. Overeating when feeling stressed, sad or bored is widespread in overweight people but often ignored.[131] Therefore, uncover and target emotional eating by using a diary similar to the one in Chapter 10. In this diary, however, note down emotions along with food and drink consumed.

Constipation

Just as carrying extra body weight places pressure on the bladder, being constipated also compresses it, which can lead to urgency and frequency. A team of researchers in Japan studied the co-occurrence of constipation and the severity of symptoms in 145 women with OAB. Over 40% of the women suffered from constipation as well as OAB, and in those with both problems, OAB symptoms were worse.[132] This connection between constipation and OAB was particularly troublesome for women who had 'wet' OAB – that is, experienced incontinence as part of the condition, as opposed to dry OAB.

What complicates matters for people with conditions like OAB who are prescribed antimuscarinic medication (Chapter 12, page 132) is that these drugs have constipation as one of their side effects. One in five people stop taking this type of medicine due to side effects,[133] which is not surprising if some of the side effects cause symptoms that can worsen the initial problem. Therefore, if you are constipated either before or during treatment for bladder symptoms, talk to your doctor. Newer kinds of antimuscarinic medicines cause less constipation than their older counterparts, and there are also other options these days, such as skin patch drugs which are detailed in the next chapter.

How do I deal with constipation?

If you have a pre-existing condition, such as a bladder problem, do discuss any over-the-counter medicines you want to try for constipation first with your doctor or pharmacist.

Also, follow the fluid intake advice above, especially if you've been limiting the amount you drink because of bladder symptoms. Even mild dehydration can cause constipation.[134] As we've just seen, both concentrated urine and constipation can aggravate the bladder, triggering symptoms. Therefore, dealing with constipation is an important aspect of tackling bladder problems for many people.

Laxatives

If you decide to take laxatives you'll need to drink more water than usual. Bulk-forming laxatives increase the amount of material in the gut, and in doing so absorb large amounts of fluid. While this makes it easier for faeces to pass through the gut, which in turn facilitates having a bowel movement (poo), there is a risk of becoming dehydrated. Therefore, always follow the guidance included in the product information sheet of every type of laxative for how much more you should drink while using it. Bran products and products such as ispaghula are types of bulk-forming laxative and are taken after a meal.

Stimulant laxatives differ from the above as they quicken the passage of waste matter through the gut. These take on average six to 12 hours to take effect and types include bisacodyl (e.g. Dulcolax), senna (e.g. Senokot) and sodium picosulphate (e.g. Dulcolax Pico).

Osmotic laxatives increase the proportion of water in the bowels, making stools softer and easier to pass. Lactulose and magnesium citrate are common types of osmotic laxatives which can be purchased from chemists and health food stores/online retailers, respectively. Movicol is another type of osmatic laxative that you can ask your chemist for. Some people have flatulence and stomach pain when they start taking these kinds of laxative, but these usually pass. Bear in mind it can take a few days for osmotic laxatives to work as they're not as fast-acting as stimulant laxatives.

It should also be noted that laxatives can work initially, but then become less effective over time, which is why it is better to rotate types if this may become a problem. In general, laxatives are not supposed to be used indefinitely so if you suffer from chronic constipation it would be worth following the exercise advice (below) as well as speaking to your doctor about ruling out any other causes and long-term management of bowel symptoms.

Exercise

Another way to help prevent and reduce both constipation and body weight is exercise, but this doesn't mean you must join a gym and become super-fit, as moderate exercise is best for gastrointestinal problems such as constipation.[135] Indeed, over-strenuous and exhaustive exercise can have the opposite effect, causing stomach-related problems. Nevertheless, regular and adequate exercise can help not only the bowel and bladder but also weight control. A simple 30-minute walk can regulate bowel movements and reduce the straining, incomplete defaecation (pooing) and hard stools (poos).[136] This moderate amount of physical activity has also been shown to speed up digestion and boost energy levels.

In addition, such modest exercise is just as good at helping people lose weight as high-intensity and lengthy routines.[137] Like all the lifestyle changes we've mentioned here, fitting in exercise to daily life should be a long-term (forever) plan. Therefore, to do this and make lasting change, it's important to be realistic and sensible. In every book that we've researched, the same overall tips have emerged – exclude any trigger food or drinks, reduce stress and move your body around. If you do the latter outdoors, you'll also get the benefit of topping-up your vitamin D levels. As we mentioned in Chapter 7, people with higher levels of vitamin D were less at risk of bladder cancer, so a stroll around the neighbourhood for just half an hour a day, can reduce symptoms now and protect your health in the future.

Summary and conclusion

In this chapter, we've looked at some changes that we can all make (with some support) to improve not only bladder symptoms but overall quality of life. Small adjustments in daily activities can make a big difference to health and wellbeing. This is not to say that it's easy to change the habits of a lifetime, but exercise, managing stress and tackling additional symptoms such as constipation can all be part of a wider plan to take control and tackle bladder symptoms head-on.

In the next chapter, we outline common medications used for bladder problems. As all drugs have side effects, it would be worth trying the behavioural methods (Chapter 9), the exclusion diet (Chapter 10) and the lifestyle changes in this chapter first to see how much these non-pharmacological treatments help.

Chapter 12

Medications for bladder conditions

In this chapter, we outline the various medicines used to treat some of the conditions covered so far in this book. Most of these medications will be prescribed by your general practitioner or consultant; you may want to discuss them as part of your treatment plan. However, as with most chronic conditions, there may not be a 'magic bullet' that completely eradicates all of your symptoms so we do suggest that everyone (whether with an invisible illness or not) tries relaxation techniques, pays attention to the food they eat and participates in activities that get the heart pumping. It may sound like the same old advice, but in every condition we've studied, researched and written about, these suggestions are always consistent. And of course, some of these changes are easier said than done, so take your time and think about some of the recommendations in Chapter 15.

Medications for controlling bladder contractions

Anticholinergic/antimuscarinic medication

If you've been diagnosed with overactive bladder (OAB), one of the first drug treatments a doctor will consider is called anticholinergic (or antimuscarinic) medication. This is because these drugs prevent the action of the neurotransmitter acetylcholine. As we discussed in Chapter 3, the bladder is controlled by the central nervous system. When the brain and bladder communicate, the communication signals are carried by chemical messengers called neurotransmitters. If these transmitters are blocked, any miscommunication leading to overactivity of bladder contractions, for example, can be prevented. This, in turn, should stop symptoms such as urgency and frequency. For some people with IC who have urge incontinence, anticholinergic medicines may also help control symptoms.

There are many different types of anticholinergic medicine. Your doctor will weigh up the pros and cons of each. As with any drug, there are side effects. Names of medications you may be given are:

- Fesoterodine fumarate (brand name Toviaz)
- Oxybutynin hydrochloride (brand names Cystrin, Ditropan, Lyrinel XL (modified release))
- Propiverine hydrochloride (brand name Detrunorm)
- Solifenacin succinate (brand names Vesicare, Tolterodine, Detrusitol, Detrusitol XL (modified release))
- Trospium chloride (brand name Regurin)

Medications can substantially help some people with bladder problems. However, if your symptoms change or worsen, or you suffer from side effects, go back to your doctor as Denny did to see if the dosage or type of tablet might be reviewed:

I went to the doctor and he gave me Vesicare tablets. They did help at first. I just took one tablet and it was incredible – I wasn't having to go to the loo all the time. But then I went back to the doctor's when I felt they weren't so helpful and he put me on two – so now I'm taking two, so a higher dosage and it's better than it was but not as good as when I first started taking the tablets.

Denny

Options with fewer side effects

Some people find the side effects of taking anticholinergic medications quite difficult. Therefore, there is an option of a skin patch and also ways to deal with the dry mouth (see below) caused by the drugs.

Transdermal oxybutynin

Instead of taking anticholinergic medicine in a tablet, oxybutynin also comes in a skin patch (transdermal oxybutynin, brand name Kentera). When drugs are administered via the skin, they're absorbed directly into the bloodstream and so essentially bypass the digestive system and liver. This means that side effects, such as nausea and constipation, may be reduced. Therefore, for people who suffer severely from such side effects, a skin patch may be a better option in terms of treatment for OAB.

Dealing with dry mouth caused by anticholinergic medication

Dry mouth is one of the most common side effects reported from the use of anticholinergic medication. This is because the mechanism of the drug not only affects the bladder, but also other parts of the body, including the salivary glands, colon and smooth muscle of the eye. Consequently, in addition to dry mouth, people can experience constipation and blurred vision, amongst other side effects. (For every medicine you take, the drug's patient information sheet will contain a full list of side effects and the proportion of people that are known to suffer from each effect – if you can't find this info sheet ask your pharmacist for a new copy as information online may be inaccurate.) Having a dry mouth persistently may lead to a burning or scalding sensation, oral infections (particularly candidiasis) and periodontal disease. Some people find the side effects of anticholinergic medication too difficult and unpleasant to cope with, but there are some things you can do to limit a dry mouth, which may be a better option if the treatment is ameliorating bladder symptoms. These are:

- Sip small amounts of cool water throughout the day
- Suck pieces of ice
- Don't smoke – either cigarettes, cigars or pipes (vaping may also make a dry mouth worse)
- Avoid foods high in sugar
- Reduce caffeine intake
- Chew sugar-free gum or sugar-free fruit pastilles to stimulate saliva production (e.g. Salivix pastilles)
- Practise good oral hygiene by brushing twice a day and flossing teeth once a day; also attend regular dental check-ups every six months
- Use a saliva substitute such as Aquoral, Biotène Oralbalance gel, AS Saliva Orthana Spray or Xerotin.

If the dry mouth continues and becomes overwhelming for you, speak to your doctor and make sure the anticholinergic medicine you've been prescribed is one that limits dry mouth – for instance, modified or extended-release preparations of these medications reduce dry mouth in some patients, making the treatment more tolerable.[138]

How effective are anticholinergic medications for the treatment of bladder conditions?

A comprehensive review of anticholinergic drugs, for people with OAB, concluded that this type of medication is effective, safe and well tolerated and also improves overall quality of life in those that use it.[139] Anticholinergics significantly reduce the number of times those with OAB need to empty their bladders and lessen the number of accidents they have. Over a 12-week period, 72% of people taking the brand Tolterodine suffered less urge incontinence, which meant that they reduced their use of incontinence pads.[140] However, there is controversy over this type of drug's benefit for interstitial cystitis (IC) and so alternative treatments (below) may be more appropriate for this condition (unsurprisingly considering the different potential causes of IC, see Chapter 6).

Betmiga (mirabegron)

Betmiga (of which the active ingredient is mirabegron) works in a different way from anticholinergic medicines as it stimulates beta-3 receptors in the bladder muscles, rather than preventing the action of acetylcholine. Beta-3 receptors are situated on the surface of muscle cells in the bladder wall and when they are triggered/stimulated, the bladder relaxes. This in turn allows the bladder to fill more, but it doesn't affect the voiding (weeing) process (see Chapter 3, for the two phases of micturition). Mirabegron does have some notable side effects, however, including hypertension, urinary tract infection and increased frequency of the common cold.[141] However, mirabegron is an effective treatment for OAB and its side effects are less likely to occur than those of anticholinergic drugs, which can help people to stay on the treatment they need.[142]

Botox injections for OAB and IC

Although Botox is best known as a way to reduce facial wrinkles, it has many medical uses also. Botox is the commercial name for botulinum toxin, which is a neurotoxin produced by the bacterium *Clostridium botulinum*. Botox works by blocking the communication between nerve cells and muscle cells. It influences numerous neurotransmitters involved with bladder function, which means if anticholinergic medicine does not work for a patient, or if the side effects of the drug are too difficult for someone to cope with, it could be a good option.[143] In this sense, Botox would more likely be offered after other, less invasive, treatments (i.e. oral medications) have been tried.

How effective is Botox for the treatment of bladder conditions?

Botox has been used for both OAB and IC. Research has

shown that in up to 80% of people with OAB, Botox treatment completely eradicated their symptoms.[144] In those with IC, over 70% of people saw improvements in their symptoms one month after the injections.[145] Therefore, Botox appears to be a good alternative or additional treatment for patients with bladder conditions who do not respond to first-line medications.

How is Botox administered?

For people with bladder dysfunction, Botox is injected directly into the bladder. To do this, a doctor will pass a cystoscope through the urethra, so, this procedure is very much like a cystoscopy as outlined in Chapter 8 (page 86). Anaesthetic gel will first be administered to numb the urethra so you shouldn't feel any pain – this may just sting a little. Then, sterile water is used to fill the bladder so that the doctor can see exactly where to place the injections of Botox. Between 10 and 30 individual injections are usually given in one procedure and this takes around half an hour from start to finish. The beneficial effects of the Botox, which include reduced urgency, frequency and urge incontinence, typically last six to nine months, but for some people symptom relief can be even longer. It takes anywhere from three days to three weeks for the effects to start. By four to six week after the injections, the results of Botox should be at their best. For some people, Botox will be given in addition to the medications we've already described; for others, it may be provided on its own.

Will there be any after effects following Botox?

As the procedure uses a cystoscope, the after effects can be similar to those after a cystoscopy (need to go to the toilet straight after, small amounts of blood in the urine, risk of infection, etc). In addition to these, the substance can also lead to flu-like symptoms, pain and muscle weakness. These symptoms are generally mild and pass in a couple of weeks. Over-the-counter medicines can be used to relieve pain if needed.

What are the risks associated with Botox?

The most common risk associated with this treatment for bladder problems is water retention.[146] Approximately one in six people will experience difficulty in going to the toilet after the Botox injections. This is why everyone who undergoes this procedure is shown how to self-catheterise. The passing of a catheter through the urethra to drain urine from the bladder is needed two to three times a day by people who do experience retention. However, as the effects of the Botox start to diminish, so does the need to self-catheterise – in other words, this side effect is not permanent, and is seen more in people with neurological conditions (multiple sclerosis or spinal problems) than in those with bladder issues alone.

Medications for nocturia and bedwetting

Desmopressin

Our bodies produce a chemical messenger called vasopressin which tells our kidneys how much water to pass out in urine. If less water is passed from the kidneys, urine will be more concentrated and the amount of fluid passed into the bladder will be less. Vasopressin is also known as the antidiuretic hormone (or ADH) and can be manufactured synthetically for people who don't produce or release enough of this vital hormone. The artificial ADH is called desmopressin and is licensed under the brand names DDAVP, DesmoMelt, Desmospray, Desmotabs, Noqdirna and Octim.

Because desmopressin regulates the volume of urine that is passed to the bladder, it can be used for night-time frequency (nocturia) and bedwetting (nocturnal enuresis). By having a smaller volume of urine in the bladder, the bladder is less likely to empty involuntarily. Desmopressin can be prescribed for children who struggle with bedwetting and is also used for people with a certain type of diabetes (cranial diabetes insipidus) wherein the brain produces or releases less ADH/vasopressin than required. Different brands of desmopressin are prescribed for different medical conditions – your doctor will discuss which brand may be the best option for you if he thinks a synthetic ADH is something that might alleviate your symptoms.

Pain medicines

Some analgesics (pain relief medicines) stop the pain signals that go to the brain, but they do not tackle the cause of the problem. Other painkillers have anti-inflammatory properties so they can address the source of the pain, to some degree at least. The most common analgesics available in chemists are paracetamol and ibuprofen. If you have pain around the urethra, analgesic creams can be used to relieve discomfort by numbing the area. Your pharmacist will be able to suggest a suitable cream for this. If your pain is so severe that it stops you doing your usual daily activities, speak to your doctor as s/he may want to give you a prescription-only analgesic. However, be aware that long-term use of painkillers can lead to addiction, constipation and other physical and psychological symptoms. Therefore, if pain is an ongoing and constant symptom, ask your doctor about local pain clinics which are usually led by psychologists who offer non-drug techniques, such as cognitive behaviour therapy (CBT), which can be an effective way to control pain without the side effects.

Antidepressants

Your doctor may suggest you take a specific type of antidepressant, not because you're depressed, but because some antidepressants also act as a pain reliever or target the nerves that control the muscles involved in weeing.

Amitriptyline

Amitriptyline is used to treat chronic pain in many conditions, including arthritis, back/neck pain, fibromyalgia, chronic headaches and peripheral neuropathy. For pain, tricyclic antidepressants are usually given in lower doses than for the treatment of depression or anxiety, but some people do find this dose lifts their mood. It usually takes around two to six weeks for amitriptyline to start reducing pain and improving mood. It can also help people sleep and relax their muscles, which may therefore limit the number of times someone needs to get up and go to the toilet during the night. However, because this drug has a sedative effect, it can cause daytime sleepiness and grogginess, so your doctor will want to discuss these and other side effects with you to make sure it's right for you. Other side effects include dry mouth, constipation and difficulty passing urine (especially in men with prostate problems), so if you have any of these symptoms already, do mention them to your doctor.

Duloxetine

Duloxetine is a type of antidepressant that interferes with some neurochemicals (serotonin and noradrenaline) in the brain. These neurochemicals are involved in sending messages from the brain to the pelvic floor muscles. Hence, by taking this type of antidepressant, the altered signals can help the pelvic floor muscles contract more strongly, which in turn may help prevent stress incontinence leaks in women. It is generally recommended that pelvic floor exercises are tried first. For women who do not want to go through surgery for their incontinence, this drug may be beneficial. In a study spanning four geographical continents, including Europe and North America, duloxetine was found to reduce stress incontinence better than a dummy (placebo) pill.[147] However, 17% of the women taking this medication experienced side effects such as nausea so severely that they stopped using this as a treatment for bladder leaks. Nevertheless, in the women overall, quality of life improved after taking duloxetine for 12 weeks.

Antihistamines (for IC)

It may seem strange that medicines used to treat hayfever and other allergies are used for IC, but this relates to the inflammation theory of IC (see Chapter 6, page 66). When histamines are released as part of our immune response, they cause inflammation so suppressing their action may have beneficial effects for inflammatory conditions.

Histamines are produced when the body thinks a foreign, and damaging, substance has invaded. They bind to receptors which trigger an allergic reaction with the classic allergy symptoms, such as sneezing, wheezing, congestion, itching, headache, increased heart rate and stomach cramps. Antihistamines work by blocking these receptors, thus preventing the 'invasion' message getting through.

Hydroxyzine

One type of antihistamine used to treat IC contains the active ingredient hydroxyzine (brand names Atarax and Ucerax). These types of antihistamine are also commonly used to relieve the itching caused by hives and eczema and control anxiety symptoms in adults. Hydroxyzine controls symptoms by blocking the receptors that produce allergic reactions. As this is a sedating antihistamine, it is likely to make you feel sleepy.

Cimetidine

Cimetidine (brand name Tagamet) is traditionally a heartburn remedy and used to treat gastro-oesophageal reflux disease (GERD) and stomach ulcers. Other uses include the reduction of hives and itching and the treatment of viral warts. Cimetidine works in a different way from atarax as it not only modifies an allergic reaction but also reduces stomach acid. The understanding with regard to IC is that cimetidine also blocks the effect of histamine on bladder cells, hence controlling symptoms.

The above antihistamine medicines require a prescription but some over-the-counter antihistamines, such as loratadine (e.g. Clarityn) and cetirizine (e.g. Benadryl, Piriteze, Zirtek), may also be helpful to control IC symptoms.

Rebuilding the bladder wall – Elmiron

Elmiron is the brand name for pentosan polysulphate sodium, which is the first oral medication developed specifically for IC. One explanation for this condition is that the bladder wall becomes more permeable (see Chapter 6, page 67), meaning that irritants can pass through the outer layer causing pain and urgency. It is thought that Elmiron works by repairing the cells of the bladder wall so that it becomes protected from aggravating substances. In a study of 41 women with IC, those taking this medicine for 12 weeks had a 46% improvement in their symptoms, which also boosted their overall quality of life.[148] Your doctor can prescribe Elmiron 'off-label', meaning it's up to the doctor's discretion to prescribe this drug as it's not licensed in many countries, including the UK, for use in IC yet (more research needs to be done for a licence to be granted). Side effects of this drug include diarrhoea, headache, nausea, rash, alopecia and rectal bleeding, so these will all need to be discussed with your doctor to see if Elmiron is right for you. Also, as Elmiron is a blood thinner (used for the prevention of blood clots), bleeding and bruising may increase when taking it. Nevertheless, it's heartening that new pharmacological treatments are being established for IC as there may be more than one cause of the condition.

Intravesical medications (for IC)

Intravesical simply means 'situated in the bladder'. These medicines are directly inserted into the bladder via a small catheter.

After having the cystoscopy and then being diagnosed with a chronically inflamed bladder (later I was told interstitial cystitis), I was given a liquid medicine called Uracyst. I was a bit shocked when the consultant said it had to go directly into the bladder with a catheter, but I was so very desperate for relief that I didn't think too much about it. At first I had to travel all the way to the hospital every week for the 'injections' as I called them. Nurses at the clinic 'injected' the Uracyst and sometimes it was painful as I found it hard to relax. It's a very strange thing how tight those muscles can be and you do not even know it! After six weeks, I only had to have the 'bladder installations' (which is what they're actually called!) once a month and then the nurse taught me how to do it myself. I was so relieved (again!) to be able to use the catheters at home as the hospital was quite a journey for me – which is of course very hard with IC. Also, you can't pee for at least an hour so the medicine can work so it was a case of sitting round the hospital, which isn't wonderful. But I really can't complain at all. After over a decade of being fobbed off I finally had a solution. It took about two years to completely settle down but now I'm completely fine. I would go so far as saying I'm 'cured', which to me is nothing short of a miracle.

Anne

There are different types of intravesical medications, which work in slightly different ways. As mentioned above, Uracyst is a bladder installation that replenishes the bladder lining with a protective coating, effectively making it 'waterproof' again. Cystistat, Gepan instill, Hyacyst and iAluRil work in similar ways but with differing compositions (different amounts of active ingredients).

DMSO (dimethyl sulphoxide) is a bladder instillation that is thought to be anti-inflammatory, which is why it's been shown to help with the symptoms of IC; it is unlicensed for the treatment of IC in the UK, but it is available from 'special-order' manufacturers or specialist importing companies.

Cystilieve is also a special-order treatment that's made out of lidocaine (an anaesthetic drug) and simple sodium bicarbonate. Your doctor can order these products if s/he thinks they may help your condition.

Another special-order preparation is Parson's Solution which also contains lidocaine to immediately control pain, combined with high-dose heparin. Heparin is both anti-inflammatory and mimics the activity of the bladder lining, which can limit further irritation, thus allowing the bladder to heal. Parson's Solution is designed to work fast and research has shown that up to 94% of patients report immediate symptom relief. Altogether, 80% of those who experienced IC reduction had symptom relief for a further two weeks after treatment; however, how long the treatment lasts does vary between people.[149]

Summary and conclusion

In this chapter, we've looked at some medications that your doctor may prescribe to treat bladder problems and symptoms. This is not an exhaustive list but rather a discussion of the most commonly recommended drug treatments for prevalent issues such as incontinence, OAB and IC. All medications have side effects, however, so we, as researchers and fellow patients who have tried many therapies in the past, would suggest that non-pharmacological treatments are considered as well. These can be used either alongside medications or as a first port of call in tackling bladder problems. Whatever you decide to do, talk openly with your doctor so that s/he can keep up to date with your progress and advise if an alternative treatment would be worth introducing into your overall management plan.

Chapter 13

Other medical devices and surgery

The previous chapter looked at medicines, either taken by mouth or directly inserted via a catheter into the bladder, used to prevent, control or – in some cases – put an end to bladder symptoms. Whilst these can be very effective for some people, for others, they may not stop urgency, frequency and incontinence, and/or the side effects of the drugs may be more severe than a person can comfortably live with. Therefore, doctors have developed alternative, non-drug treatments to help reduce bladder symptoms. Some of these techniques are quite invasive and involve surgery and so pose the same risks as any surgical procedure, including infection and pain. Therefore, we would always suggest trying the dietary changes (Chapter 10) and behavioural treatments, such as pelvic floor muscle exercises (Chapter 9), first as a foundation for bladder health.

Catheterisation

As we've mentioned in Chapter 8 (investigations), a catheter is a thin tube that is inserted into the urethra to drain urine from the bladder. While most people know what a catheter is, the thought of using one can seem distressing.

When the nurse first mentioned catheters, I freaked out inside. Even though I was only using it to give myself the medicine (bladder installation), I felt like an old woman. But when the treatment started to work and I got my life back, I soon forgot about feeling like that.

Anne

Catheters aren't only used to administer medication however; catheters can be used as a form of treatment in themselves, for instance if there's nerve damage or weakness in the bladder, if there's an obstruction that's affecting the urethra or for incontinence and urine retention.

Intermittent catheters

Intermittent catheters are used temporarily through the day to empty the bladder – some people only need to do this once a day, but this depends on a person's circumstances and habits. Below Hannah describes how using intermittent catheterisation helped to restore normal life following the birth of her first child.

The thought of sticking something into my wee hole was horrendous. But it really isn't all that bad. I managed to do it straight away with the help of a mirror and I was surprised by how easy and painless it was. Of course, I was upset that it had come to this and the thought of doing this in a public toilet worried me. But it gave me freedom and I was able to go for short walks with my partner and baby whereas before I found the in-dwelling catheters too uncomfortable to leave the house for long periods.

Hannah

This type of self-catheterisation, even if it at first seems unpleasant, can give some people back control over their bodies and lives. Hannah subsequently recovered and no longer needed to catheterise but others may need to do this on an ongoing basis.

In-dwelling catheters

As Hannah mentioned, she was offered the choice of an in-dwelling catheter, which stays inserted into the urethra for days or weeks at a time. For some people, this is a more appropriate option if symptoms such as overflow incontinence are particularly severe or if self-catheterisation is found to be difficult. In in-dwelling catheterisation, a bag collects the wee and it is this that is emptied. This type of catherisation can be more convenient also as it avoids the need to continually insert a catheter. However, a catheter that sits in place for any length of time holds a risk of blockage with sediment and of infection.

Surgical procedures

Some people with bladder issues may opt for surgical procedures, usually when diet, exercise and medications have given only limited benefit. All surgical procedures carry risks so the pros and cons of each option will need to be discussed carefully with your specialist. For example, for women who would like to have children, surgery may not be the best option as the treatment may fail following pregnancy and childbirth. However, surgical methods are possibilities that you may want to explore if your quality of life has been adversely affected due to bladder problems.

Tape procedures

For some women with stress incontinence, the insertion of a length of specially developed plastic tape behind the urethra may help prevent leaks. The surgeon will make an incision in the vaginal wall, with either end of the piece of tape attached internally to the tops of the inner thigh (known as 'transobturator tape procedure', or TOT) or the abdomen (which is called a 'retropubic tape procedure' or 'tension-free vaginal tape procedure'; TVT).[150]

This is essentially like having an extra 'hammock' inside the body to hold the urethra in its normal position and keep it closed when laughing, coughing, sneezing etc. The pelvic floor muscles would usually do this job, but sometimes, because of damage to or weakness in these muscles, the urethra sags (see Chapter 9, page 101). After one year of TOT surgery, researchers in Belgium at the Erasmus Hospital found 80% of a group of 120 women with stress incontinence were completely dry and a further 12% had improved greatly. These women said they could be more active, had a better view of themselves and also had better sex lives than before the procedure.

An even longer-scale study of TVT showed that 90% of women who had this procedure had remained symptom-free 11.5 years after surgery.[151] Only 3% of the women thought the procedure had been a failure. However, with both types of tape procedure, the plastic tape can shift within the body and you may need an additional procedure to remove or adjust it. A small proportion of women (5-10%) report pain on going to the toilet, needing to go more often and having feelings of urgency. Urine retention (not being able to wee) and infections may also occur but these are even less common, found in 1-5% of patients. These and any other possible side effects would be discussed with you by the specialist before the procedure.

Tape procedures are not suitable for men.

Colposuspension

Colposuspension, sometimes known as Burch colposuspension after the surgeon John Burch who first outlined the procedure, is a technique that lifts tissue around the junction of the bladder and urethra (sometimes called the neck of the bladder). Once this tissue is lifted, it is stitched into place behind the pubic bone, providing additional support for women with stress incontinence. There are two kinds of colposuspension, which differ in their invasiveness: open colposuspension is carried out through a large incision, whereas laparoscopic colposuspension involves keyhole surgery that only requires a small incision. Both types of procedure are effective in treating stress incontinence, but the keyhole surgery allows for faster recovery as it's not such a major operation.[152] However, in the UK, keyhole colposuspension may not be available in all areas as it needs to be carried out by an experienced laparoscopic surgeon. Also, side effects such as not being able to empty the bladder fully, urgency and frequency, infection and painful sex have been reported.[153]

Like tape procedures, colposuspension is not suitable for men.

Sling procedures

Sling procedures are similar to tape techniques but here the 'sling' can be made out of material from your own body (autologous sling), donated from someone else (allograft sling) or from an animal such as a pig or cow (xenograft sling). There are also synthetic sling materials that can be used, but the long-term effects of these are less well known.

This procedure can be used in both women and men who have stress incontinence, although it is more commonly used for women and most male cases have so far mainly been in research studies, not everyday medical practice.

Other surgical procedures

Artificial urinary sphincter

For men with stress incontinence, fitting an artificial sphincter may be appropriate. This technique is rarely carried out on women, however. The sphincter consists of muscles that stop urine seeping from the bladder into the urethra. The artificial type consists of three parts, as shown in Figure 8:

- a 'cuff' that is circular in shape and fitted around the urethra – when filled with sterile saline solution the cuff closes the urethra so wee can't escape – think of the cuff as a stop valve;
- a pump that sits in the scrotum and controls the action of the cuff by regulating the flow of liquid to and from the cuff;
- a balloon that is placed in the abdomen that holds the liquid that is pumped in and out of the cuff – this acts as a reservoir to house the liquid which either opens or closes the cuff via the pump.

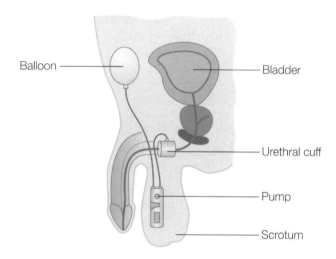

Figure 8: The components of an artificial sphincter

The procedure to fit these components can cause some bleeding, but this shouldn't last. The bigger issue with artificial sphincters is that they can erode or the pump mechanism can fail. Therefore, some patients may need a further operation to remove the damaged device – over a quarter of people have been shown to require an additional procedure, but this should be weighed up against the 86% of men who have reported becoming 'dry' with the artificial sphincter.[154]

Augmentation cystoplasty

A very small proportion of people with bladder problems may be offered an augmentation cystoplasty. This procedure enlarges the bladder by taking a piece of tissue (usually from the bowel) and attaching it to the bladder wall and is therefore most likely to be considered for people with small capacity in their bladders. Its use in people with IC is quite controversial but for those with urge incontinence, there is more support for its use.[155] Because some patients have trouble emptying their bladders normally after the operation, only people who are comfortable using a catheter will be considered for this treatment. However, it may be an option for people with conditions such as spinal cord injury or multiple sclerosis.

Urinary diversion

Urinary diversion is rarely used and only for patients who have tried, or cannot use, all other treatments. In this procedure, the normal structures of the urinary system are bypassed and an alternative opening is created to drain urine from the body. For instance, the tubes connecting the kidneys to the bladder (the ureters – see Chapter 2, page 22) can be redirected so that they circumvent the bladder altogether (this is known as an 'ileal conduit diversion'). Wee then passes through a hole called a stoma and is collected in a bag that sits outside the body (the stoma bag).

Other types of urinary diversion create another pouch within the body that is then emptied with a catheter (e.g. Mitrofanoff continent urinary diversion). In general, people who have the latter procedure have a better quality of life than those who require a stoma.[156]

Urethral bulking agents

For women, a substance called a bulking agent can be injected into the walls of the urethra to, in effect, make them bigger. This means it's easier for the urethra to stay closed, which in turn reduces stress incontinence. The substance used to bulk the urethra walls varies from synthetic materials to animal collagen or transplanted tissue from the patient. All types of bulking agent work about as well as the others and are safe and well tolerated.[157] As the substance can be injected during a cystoscopy (Chapter 8, page 86), this is a somewhat less intrusive procedure compared to slings and tapes. But there are concerns over the durability of the bulking agents and for many this is a less effective long-term option for the treatment of stress incontinence. This procedure isn't as successful in men so unlikely to be offered to male patients.[158]

Neuromodulation therapy

'Neuro' means 'relating to nerves or the nervous system'; modulation relates to modifying or controlling something. Thus neuromodulation therapies are treatments that target the nerves involved with bladder function (see Chapter 3), specifically in conditions such as overactive bladder syndrome (OAB) where the nerves seem to be over-firing. These may be particularly useful for people that find it hard to tolerate medication. There are two main types of neuromodulation therapy:

- Sacral nerve stimulation (SNS) therapy – Here the sacral nerves which are involved in the control of many muscles relating to bladder function, including the bladder itself, urethral sphincters and the pelvic floor muscles, are stimulated;
- Percutaneous tibial nerve stimulation (PTNS) – This is an indirect method of stimulating the nerves that control the bladder and pelvic floor as it targets the tibial nerve. The

tibial nerve runs down the leg to the ankle but originates from the same area as the sacral nerve.

How does neuromodulation therapy work?

Small electrodes that emit electrical signals are placed under the skin, near the bladder, in a device called a 'neurostimulator' which is very like a heart pacemaker. The device has a thin 'lead' attached to it which is an insulated wire, so that the electrical impulses can be tweaked by a doctor. This may sound like something out of a sci-fi or horror novel, but the procedure is safe and can be effective for people with conditions such as incontinence, IC and OAB where no other treatment has worked.

In SNS the device is inserted in a pocket in the patient's lower abdomen. SNS is first tried on an outpatient basis in the doctor's office with the implantation of a test lead. If the trial treatment is successful, the patient is scheduled for inpatient surgery.

In percutaneous tibial nerve stimulation (PTNS), a small, thin needle is inserted into the ankle which is connected to the device, so it's much less intrusive than SNS.

What does neuromodulation therapy feel like?

The electrical signals are mild so it doesn't feel like a severe electric shock; in fact, most people say it feels like a gentle tingling or pulsating sensation around their pelvic area or foot, depending on the type of procedure.

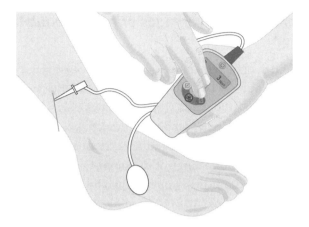

Figure 9: Equipment for PTNS

How effective is neuromodulation therapy?

In 59% of people with urge incontinence, SNS halved their number of leaks per day and these results continued when the patients were assessed three years after treatment. Forty-six per cent of people didn't experience incontinence at all after the SNS. For people who needed to use the loo often and with urgency, 56% had a substantial improvement two years after the procedure. For a year and a half following the SNS, those with retention had a more than 50% reduction in the amount of wee that was drained from their catheters.[159]

In the Overactive Bladder Innovative Therapy trial, PTNS was compared with drug treatment (tolterodine) in 100 people with OAB. Almost 80% of those who had PTNS said they were either symptom-free or greatly improved, whereas only 55% on the medication saw symptom relief.[160] In the same trial, researchers looked at how durable the treatment was over a year and found that the improvements in the number of times people had to go to the toilet both in the day and at night, urge incontinence, and the amount of wee that they could pass each time, were all sustained.[161]

What are the disadvantages of neuromodulation therapy?

The main risk of SNS therapy is infection because it is a surgical procedure. Your doctor may prescribe antibiotics to limit the risk of infection in the area where the device was inserted and you may need pain relief while the incision wound heals. Some people (about a third) may need another operation to readjust the lead.[162] Pain and feelings of discomfort can follow after the procedure but these are often outweighed by the benefits of being dry and symptom-free. As PTNS is minimally invasive, the risks are much lower; however, because this is a newer method, there isn't as much research about it so it's less likely to be offered as a routine treatment.

Summary and conclusion

In this chapter we have outlined a number of devices and surgical treatments for people with incontinence and bladder conditions. There is quite a range of options for those who do not find effective relief from diet, exercise and medication. However, many of these procedures are invasive and life changing and therefore can adversely affect quality of life so may only be considered if all other alternatives have been exhausted. In the next chapter, we explore treatments that come from complementary and alternative medicine (CAM).

Chapter 14

Complementary and alternative medicine (CAM)

The trend towards the increased use of CAM is patient-driven and reflects the change in values perceived by patients toward conventional medical treatment. Furthermore, the need for personal control, the perceived safety of a 'natural' product and a search for potential curative therapies when conventional treatments are expected to offer little benefit has driven the surge in the popularity of CAM.

Yiannis Philippou and colleagues, East Surrey Hospital, UK[163]

This chapter outlines the evidence for relevant treatments within the field of complementary and alternative medicine (or 'CAM'), including acupuncture, hypnotherapy and supplements. From data collected in 2002, it was found that 62% of US adults over 18 had tried some form of CAM in the past year.[164] There are many thousands of products and treatments on the market for all sorts of health problems – from general fatigue to cancer – and so it can be very difficult to navigate this area. Therefore, in this chapter we focus on the evidence base for CAM therapies so that you may make informed choices about whether to try such alternatives.

Research in CAM

Although there are many herbs and preparations suggested for bladder problems, it is actually quite difficult to find studies which have found positive results in humans. This may be because these types of treatments do not effectively treat bladder conditions, but it also may be due to inadequate research funding. High-quality studies cost many thousands, if not millions, of pounds and so without significant financial backing a research study may be of poor quality or not happen at all. It's often difficult for alternative and complementary therapies to attract this kind of funding so it's worth just noting that a dearth of studies does not necessarily mean that we won't in the future find adjunct treatments for bladder problems. But for now, this chapter focuses on the evidence we have to date.

Why do people use CAM, then?

Some bladder conditions are difficult to diagnose (e.g. interstitial cystitis – IC) and it can take many years for a correct diagnosis to be made. You may have experienced this or are still trying to find an answer for your symptoms – this is not uncommon.

> My doctor said that I was imagining things, that I had no bladder problems! She did not say that to me, but to my mother and she started to be sceptical of me, and my condition. I can't say I blame the doctor or my mother; they did the best they have known. But I felt humiliated and crazy. I started to doubt my own self. And so I decided to pretend that my problem no longer existed. I was quiet for nine years, I was managing alone, did not drink too much, I avoided some foods... I did all kinds of things just to make my condition better.
>
> *Martina*

People can also feel disbelieved or that their symptoms are not legitimised by health professionals, as Martina mentions above. This sense of delegitimisation can lead to additional problems and people often feel isolated and alone, not only with their health issues but in general. Martina spent nine years concealing her bladder issues and only sought help again when the symptoms became utterly unbearable. During this time, she tried a number of self-help and CAM methods. We have found this pattern in many of the invisible illnesses we've studied over the years – including IBS, CFS/ME and mal de debarquement syndrome (MdDS). In other words, people with invisible illnesses, and especially with those in which there is no clear or agreed upon cause (as is the case with IC), seek out non-orthodox treatments not only for symptom alleviation but because CAM therapies tend to take a more integrative approach. This approach allows for multiple explanatory models (that is, how both patients and practitioners make sense of health problems) that in turn lead to patients feeling more listened to and legitimised. This can be very important as we know that stigma is directly related to quality of life and functioning in many conditions.

Acupuncture

Acupuncture was originally a type of traditional Chinese treatment, where the practitioner inserted fine needles into various points on the body in order to stimulate certain areas (acupuncture points). It was thought that when people became ill or had pain, the body's vital energy (qi) was being blocked. The way to release the energy was by inserting needles in the correct places on the body, which would restore balance to the system. Western practitioners tend not to accept the traditional explanation regarding energy blockages.

We now believe that acupuncture works by reducing inflammation, encouraging the release of endorphins (yet another type of neurotransmitter that can block the release of pain signals) and calming the mind. It is a safe treatment. The only side effects that have been reported are pain at the place

where the needles are inserted, and lethargy (tiredness), both of
which are short-lasting.

Arroll and Dancey[165]

Acupuncture is now accepted as a useful tool for treating pain, and has been used for chronic pain in osteoarthritis, hypertension, tinnitus, headache, Tourette's syndrome, PTSD, anxiety, depression and many other conditions, including bladder dysfunction.

There are also studies of acupuncture in rats, horses, dogs and cows. Many of these studies show good effects of acupuncture, and so it is reasonable to think that humans might benefit from acupuncture as well. In fact, Narda Robinson of the Center for Comparative and Integrative Pain Medicine, College of Veterinary Medicine and Biomedical Sciences in Colorado, says:

Between animal and human medicine there is no dividing line
– nor should there be. The object is different but the experience
obtained constitutes the basis of all medicine... the need for
a holistic, collaborative approach – one strategy to better
understand and address the contemporary health issues created
by the convergence of human, animal and environmental
domains is the concept of One Health.[166]

In relation to humans, researchers in the James Paget University Hospital in Norfolk discussed a case where a 49-year-old woman who had bladder problems was treated with acupuncture.[167] Her key symptoms were urgency and increased frequency, primary symptoms of OAB. She had been having other treatments for 18 months which helped, but she was still having symptoms. It took around six treatment sessions with acupuncture before she noticed improvements in her bladder symptoms and eight sessions before she had no other episodes of OAB symptoms.

Researchers in China assessed the effectiveness of acupuncture in 240 women with OAB.[168] Altogether 118 were randomly assigned to have a weekly acupuncture treatment, and the other 122 women were given a pharmacological treatment for four weeks. The researchers took information from them on urgency, incontinence, frequency (how often they had a wee) and how often they got up in the night to wee. They found that both groups had significant decreases in their OAB symptoms.

Researchers in Norway treated women with recurrent cystitis with acupuncture. They stated that for most of the women, their bladder problems improved, and they had more energy, reduced stress levels, and better sleep.[169] Researchers in Japan found that patients who had to get up in the night to void their bladders improved significantly; their bladder capacity improved, on average, from 201 ml before treatment to 334 ml afterwards.[170]

This indicates that it might be worth trying acupuncture for bladder dysfunction.

Hypnotherapy

Hypnotherapy has been found to be effective for many different conditions. A hypnotherapist will carry out exercises that lead to your feeling extremely relaxed. As Michael Sealey, a hypnotherapist (search on YouTube), says, all hypnosis is self-hypnosis. You are in complete control and you can stop at any time if the technique makes you feel uncomfortable. It's important for you to know this, so that you can completely relax when the hypnotherapist starts talking to you. The hypnotherapist will talk to you steadily and calmly until you feel a sense of deep relaxation. Although hypnosis is an altered state of awareness, a bit like day-dreaming, most people find it very calming and a positive experience. Used for treating psychological and physiological problems, the technique often seems to work, but the question is 'how?'. It may be that when you are in a completely relaxed state, you are more open to suggestion.

There are many studies which have been carried out in order to see whether hypnotherapy is effective in a wide range of diseases, including asthma, headache, migraine, chronic pain and cancer. One of the most studied diseases is IBS (irritable bowel syndrome). Peter Whorwell in Manchester devised gut-directed hypnotherapy for IBS in the 1980s and since then the team has continued to do research in this area. One of its latest publications is called 'Hypnotherapy for irritable bowel syndrome: an audit of one thousand adult patients,' in which it notes that they have had much success with hypnotherapy in relation to IBS. They also say:

> Gut-focused hypnotherapy improves the symptoms of irritable bowel syndrome (IBS) with benefits being sustained for many years. Despite this, the technique has not been widely adopted by healthcare systems, possibly due to relatively small numbers in published studies and uncertainty about how it should be provided.

Miller and colleagues[171]

Some early studies demonstrated that some people with incontinence and interstitial cystitis (IC) could be helped with hypnotherapy. Economakis (2007) gave hypnotherapy to five incontinent women who had detrusor instability (DI).[172] They each completed 10 to 12 sessions of hypnotherapy over six months. All five women reported improved overall wellbeing; three were free of DI symptoms, one had improvements in urinary frequency, and one remained the same.

Green tea

Both green tea and black tea contain an antioxidant more potent than vitamins C and E,[173] which is said to help alleviate inflammation. Green tea has a higher concentration of the antioxidant than black tea. We found one study which looked at green tea and bladder cancer. The authors concluded that green tea polyphenols can protect against oxidative stress/damage and bladder cell death. However, we know of no study which showed that green tea can help with bladder dysfunction.

What is 'oxidative stress'?

We need oxygen to survive as it is combined with our fuel (from food) to release energy. However, during this process damaging by-products are created, known as 'free radicals'. Free radicals are dangerous as they are unstable atoms or molecules that can strip electrons from neighbouring molecules in a bid to achieve a stable structure. This in turn can cause other molecules to become unstable and result in a domino effect that can eventually damage cells and tissues. Oxidative stress is the term used for the load that an organism must bear in the continual production of free radicals during the normal process of metabolism, in addition to environmental factors (a good example of this is tobacco smoke). Luckily we have natural defences that 'soak up' these free radicals, such as physical barriers within cells, enzymes and even substances derived from our diet like vitamins C and E which have antioxidant properties. However, when we age, and in some illnesses such as heart disease, Parkinson's disease, Alzheimer's disease and cancer, there appears to be an imbalance in our oxidative stress and antioxidant defences which can lead to ill health and symptoms.

Herbs

Gosha-jinki-gan (Japanese herbs)

Kajiwara and Mutaguchi (2008) studied 44 women who had OAB. They were given 7.5 grams of gosha-jinki-gan a day for 12 weeks. They found that over 53% were improved, 41% unchanged and 7% worsened; 9% had adverse reactions, although the authors did not include any details on what these reactions were.[174]

Horsetail

Horsetail is a herb which is supposed to act as a urinary astringent and antispasmodic, and has been used to help bladder conditions. However, we could not find any scientific studies to support this.

Honey

There are scores of scientific studies all showing how good natural honey is for our health. Honey is known to have anti-cancer effects and wide benefits for us; it is useful against tumours in relation to breast, kidney, bone and bladder cancers. It is antibacterial and anti-inflammatory – especially Manuka honey – and has a wide range of health benefits in reducing fatigue and helping with pain.

Researchers in Southampton University Hospital think that honey could have a potential use in hospital patients who have to use urinary catheters, as it could prevent infections.[175] They have found that honey's anti-inflammatory properties are stronger in dark honeys, such as Manuka. In their laboratory, they showed that diluted Manuka honey strongly inhibited the growth of bacteria but as they have only tested honey in relation to bacteria in the lab, they recognise they cannot yet say that this would happen in the human bladder; further studies outside the lab need to be done.

> *The aim of this on-going project is to lay the evidential and intellectual basis for moving towards clinical trials of topical honey as a treatment for (IC) and/or as a preventive against the sequelae of long term catheter usage by describing the distribution of mast cells in human bladders, measuring products of mast cell activation in urine and applying honey preparations to bladder-derived mast cell populations.*
>
> Emineke and colleagues

Pomegranate

Pomegranates and their juice have antimicrobial and anti-inflammatory effects which have led to the possibility of therapeutic use for many different diseases, including prostate cancer and chronic obstructive pulmonary disease. One study in 2013 found that pomegranates were useful against UTIs/cystitis, and had no harmful effects on the body.[176] Given that pomegranates *could* be useful in bladder dysfunction, again it's probably a good idea to try them.

Pumpkin seed oil

Japanese researchers Nishimura and colleagues said that they had found pumpkin seed oil was useful for treating nocturia.[177] They then carried out a study to see whether it would be useful for people with OAB. Forty-five people took 10 grams of oil per day for 12 weeks. They found that this significantly reduced the symptoms of OAB. Pumpkin seed oil can be bought easily online and in health food stores, so again, it's something worth trying.

Quercetin

Quercetin occurs naturally in apples (especially the skins), onions, chilli peppers and celery and has been shown to have anti-inflammatory properties and so may help people with IC.[178]

Selenium

Selenium is a nutrient essential to our health and it may provide some protection against bladder cancer.[179] This is because our bodies use selenium to make into selenoproteins, which have antioxidant properties (see Box on page 163). Selenium appears to be particularly beneficial for women, perhaps because men and women's bodies accumulate and excrete selenium to different degrees. However, there seems to be no evidence it will help with other bladder conditions.

Vitamin D

Researchers from Sweden – Hertting and colleagues – carried out a study that suggested a role for vitamin D in protection against UTIs/cystitis.[180] It works by stimulating the production of an antimicrobial peptide called cathelicidin. They say that if people are lacking vitamin D (and it seems that's the case for most of us, especially in winter) then having supplementation to bring vitamin D levels up to the correct levels might help prepare the body to 'mount a stronger and faster immune response once bacteria enter the bladder'.

Summary and conclusion

Overall, we have found limited evidence for the effectiveness for CAM therapies in bladder dysfunction. As mentioned at the start of the chapter, in time there will be more research studies available and so we'll have more information on other types of treatments and supplements.

If you have found something that works for you, alone or in addition to more orthodox treatment, then stick with it. In the next chapter, we complete this book with further ways to help cope with bladder conditions that can be both embarrassing and isolating.

Chapter 15

Additional tips for coping with bladder conditions

In this final chapter, we describe some practical tips for coping with leaks and the anxiety which incontinence can bring about, in addition to some more general tips that can improve the quality of life for people with all sorts of long-term illness. In fact, the guidance in this chapter on how to get a good night's sleep and ways to stop our minds running away with worries can be helpful for everyone, whether they have a health issue or not.

Incontinence products

One of the last things we want in life is to become isolated, but having bladder issues can prevent people from going out, socialising and doing activities they once enjoyed. We all need to feel safe and secure in the outside world so using incontinence products may add the extra protection to allow people to enjoy daily life without fear of noticeable leaks. Incontinence products have come a long way from 'adult nappies' and there is a range of pads and pants that are much more discreet than old-fashioned large, bulky protective wear.

Pads

Panty liners and pads can be purchased from supermarkets and chemists, but over time this can become expensive. A website specifically for health-related and innovative products called StressNoMore offers reusable pantyliners. Wellys Waterproof Panty Liners can be washed and hygienically reused (http:// www.stressnomore.co.uk/). These may also appeal to people who are concerned for the environment and don't want to use non-biodegradable products.

Pants

Just like pads, incontinence pants have also been redesigned to make them invisible under clothes. Television presenter Carol Smillie has developed a range of protective underwear after talking with her daughters about periods. Realising there was nothing on the market that looked and felt like normal knickers, she created pants with an integral leak-proof panel. The machine washable underwear known as Pretty Clever Pants look nothing like an incontinence product, and can be used for light leaks, including menstruation, post-partum bleeding or bladder problems.

> *Did you know that one in three women suffer with what I call 'laughter leaks' ? (Not incontinence, which is a very different thing!) That's why I designed Pretty Clever Pants – they're machine washable with a secret waterproof panel, to protect against life's little leaks, and worn together with your normal protection, they are the perfect back-up. When you think about it, 10 years ago, no one had a sports bra, or shape wear but who doesn't own one, or both of those, now? Even if we don't do sport! Pretty Clever Pants are another piece of smart underwear in our drawer, that solves a particular problem, like heavy periods, post maternity or stress incontinence. The triple layer technology is designed to save your blushes and give women confidence to live life to the full, without embarrassment.*
>
> Carol Smillie

Pretty Clever Pants can be bought from High Street TV: www.highstreettv.com / pretty-clever-pants-singles.html

Other types of protective underwear (for both men and women) can be found at the StressNoMore website. For men, there are boxers and briefs that can hold up to 90 ml of liquid. ProTechDry men's underwear also controls odours – we know one of the most embarrassing aspects of incontinence can be the smell so these could be a good option for lighter incontinence when out and about.

Finding and accessing toilets easily

Travelling and going to places where you're not sure if you'll be able to access a toilet quickly and easily can be frightening enough to prevent trips and fun activities. However, there are ways to make toilet access more straightforward when out and about.

Just Can't Wait toilet card

The Just Can't Wait toilet card is the same size and shape as a credit card and can be carried discreetly and used in times of need. Written on this card is a polite request to use the toilet immediately because the card holder has a condition that means they need quick access to facilities. Although the card can't guarantee universal entry to toilets, it is a generally accepted way for people with conditions such as those we've covered in this book to use a WC without delay. The card is free from the Bladder and Bowel Community and delivered within five working days when ordered online (10 days for postal orders). There is also now a Just Can't Wait Card App which includes maps to find the nearest toilets and other useful information from this organisation (£1.99; currently only available on Apple devices www.bladderandbowel.org/help-information/just-cant-wait-card/)

Toilet apps for smartphones

There are many other toilet-finder apps for both Apple devices (iPhones, iPads, etc) and other types of smartphone and tablet. Many of these are free so it would be worth trying a few and seeing which one you prefer to use and suits you best. For instance, there is the Gender Neutral Toilet Finder which was created by a trans youth group in Newcastle upon Tyne and developed by the University of Newcastle to help trans people feel more comfortable in finding public facilities.

Radar key

A Radar key is a way to access disabled toilets that are usually locked to the general public. These facilities are normally locked so that people with disabilities or bladder and bowel problems don't have to wait in a queue, so that the toilets can be kept clean and to prevent vandalism. Initially introduced by the Royal Association of Disability and Rehabilitation, hence the name RADAR, these keys are now available from Disability Rights UK through the National Key Scheme for £4.50 (www. disabilityrightsuk.org/shop/radar-key). The key gives people with health conditions independent access to over 9000 accessible toilets in the UK; regional lists of facilities in this programme can also be ordered from Disability Rights UK. However, do contact your local council first as some boroughs give Radar keys free of charge to people with health conditions.

Other organisations such as Age UK sell disabled toilet keys for a much lower price (£1.09 for an easy-turn key; £1.19 for a standard key) but these are not strictly part of the scheme (www.ageukincontinence.co.uk/incontinence-shop/toilet-aids/disabled-toilet-keys.html). There is a raft of fake Radar keys on sale over the internet but bear in mind these may not work and/or might break easily. The keys are quite bulky at over twice the size of a Yale lock key, as they were designed for people with physical impairments and also for the locks to withstand heavy use.

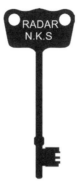

Figure 10: A Radar key for access to disabled toilets in the UK

Stress and illness

The simple fact of having a health condition is stressful. Not only do you have the everyday demands such as earning enough money, taking care of children or parents, keeping a house in order, buying and cooking food, etc, but you also have to deal with the illness itself. We can think of life as a boat ride – each demand (or stressor) is an additional bag in the boat. If we have a few of these extra bags, our boat will still sail along quite easily. In other words, we can cope with our boatload. With more extra baggage we may slow down a bit but we're still sailing. However, if the amount of extra weight from the bags becomes more than our boat can carry, we might then tip over and feel overwhelmed by it all. Having a health condition is an additional bag that we carry with us. Sometimes the weight of the bag can be lightened with treatment or self-help. For some people, the extra luggage can be taken away completely if treatment is successful. And then sometimes, even when we thought we had got rid of the bag, it gets thrown back on our boat (symptoms recur). The important point here is that for people with health conditions, because they already have the extra weight of illness to carry, the other 'bags' in their boat, such as a taxing job, energy-draining family members or even doing housework, can sink the ship. This is why we've including a stress section in this chapter

Why is it important to reduce stress?

Stress involves most bodily systems and can lead to altered microbiota, which has important health implications for people with all sorts of conditions. Stress can lead to fatigue, and worry, and be especially bad when you wake up in the night. There's no one answer to reducing stress; people have different ways of coping. Here are a few suggestions for tackling stress so that you don't have too much extra baggage on your boat weighing you down.

How to stop negative thinking patterns

What we tell ourselves is very important. If you tell yourself that you will never be able to make the journey from home to work because you will not be able to last that long before needing the toilet, then a) the worry about this will stress you and b) the worry and stress will make the feared scenario the most likely. Of course, just telling yourself you *will* get to a and b without a problem doesn't guarantee that it will happen, because you will still be focusing on this problem. To combat this type of catastrophic thinking, note down:

- how likely is it this scenario will happen?
- how awful would it be if it happened?
- how would you cope if it did happen?
- what would you say to someone else if this did happen?

By working through this logical process it is possible to feel more in control of your thought patterns, which in turn reduces stress.

Breathing exercises

Breathing deeply through the diaphragm helps to stimulate the parasympathetic nervous system. In Chapter 3, we stated that the parasympathetic nervous system is involved in bladder function and it is the part of the central nervous system that returns us to a calm state after a stressful event. Therefore, regular practice of deep breathing can be a way to manage and reduce stress, which is beneficial to both emotional and physical health. To know whether you're breathing through the diaphragm simply put one hand on your belly and one on your chest. Deep, diaphragmatic breathing occurs when the belly lifts on the inhale and dips on the exhale. If your chest is rising and falling you're breathing shallowly. We often get into this pattern over time – look at a baby to see how we all breathed in early life; his belly will move rather than his chest. The aim is to get back to this habit in day-to-day life.

Alternate nostril breathing exercise

Try to practise this alternate nostril breathing exercise (Figure 11) regularly so that when you're feeling stressed it will become second nature:

- Find a quiet place to sit and place both feet flat on the ground with your back against the chair to ground yourself.
- Lift your right hand to your face and place your thumb over the right nostril to close it (you can rest your index fingertip and middle fingertip between your eyebrows for comfort).
- Inhale slowly and deeply through the open left nostril, feeling your belly rise.
- Now use your ring finger to close the left nostril and in the next moment lift your thumb from your right nostril.
- Exhale slowly through your now open right nostril.

- Now keep your fingers in place and inhale through the right nostril.
- Next close off the right nostril again with your thumb while lifting your ring finger from the left nostril.
- Finally exhale slowly, at a steady pace though the left nostril.
- Repeat this six to 12 times, with your eyes closed if possible.

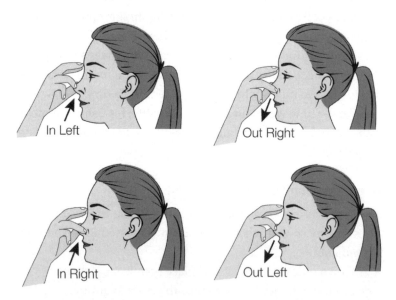

Figure 11: How to practise alternate nostril breathing

Mind-body exercises such as yoga, tai chi and Pilates also teach deep breathing methods so you may want to find a class in your local area. Some Pilates teachers also include pelvic floor exercises in their sessions – ask if this is the case so you can get the benefit of both types of instruction in one class.

Guided imagery

Guided imagery is a technique that uses the power of our minds to take us to a place of calm and relaxation. There are numerous types of guided imagery – some methods help to relieve pain, others to cope with certain fears such as flying. Guided imagery has also been used in bladder conditions such as interstitial cystitis (IC).[181] This method is for general relaxation:

- Find a peaceful place and loosen any tight clothing, remove glasses if you wear them and either sit or lie down.
- Make sure you're breathing deeply through your diaphragm (belly rising on the inhale and falling on the exhale).
- Gently close your eyes.
- Now think of your favourite type of outdoor space – this could be the beach, a forest, the countryside, mountains, anything you like.
- What can you see? The crystal blue colour of the sea; the bright green of palm trees; the blinding light of the full sun?
- Now think about the sounds you can hear – the distant crashing of the waves to shore; the light hum of music in a coastal bar; children splashing in the shallow water?
- What aromas are wafting by? Coconut oil from someone's sunscreen; sizzling meat from a restaurant up the coastline; the smell of the seaweed.
- What can you feel? Soft grains of sand in between your toes; penetrating warmth of the sun; slight moisture on your body.
- What can you taste? Subtle saltiness in the air; the sweetness of a refreshing beachside drink; charcoal at the back of your throat from a BBQ.
- The purpose here is to not just think about the beach as a remote picture, but to feel as if you are there.
- Now notice your muscles relaxing as you focus on each sense.
- Feel the calm washing over your body and mind as you

enter deeper into your chosen scene.

- When you're ready to re-enter the here and now, slowly count backwards from 10.
- On opening your eyes, you will be relaxed and feel calm, yet alert.

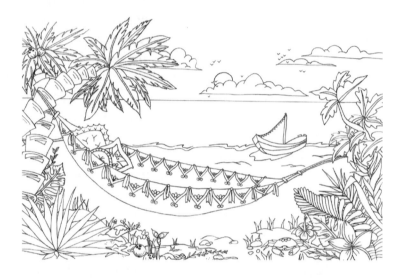

Figure 12: To de-stress, picture yourself in a place of calm beauty. (Reproduced from *Preparing for Birth: colouring your pregnancy journey* by Bridget Sheeran, illustrated by Olwyn Jennings (Hammersmith Health Books))

There are many other general stress reduction exercises that you can use, many of which can be found on internet sites, YouTube, and apps such as Headspace (www.headspace.com). There are also countless books on relaxation, mindfulness and meditation – visit your local library's mind and body or psychology section to borrow these for free to see which ones suit you.

Support of others

If we think again about the boat analogy above, if we tether our boat to others we can spread the load of life's stressors. Letting friends and family help us in practical, and emotional, ways can make living with a condition easier to cope with. This 'social support' has been researched in countless mental and physical illnesses and it's consistently been found that people who receive the help and care of others have a better overall quality of life. This is true of bladder conditions as well.[182]

Although it might be difficult, we always recommend that people talk about their condition, at least to friends and family. Although it might be embarrassing at first, talking about your condition should reduce the stigma you might feel, and ultimately, it benefits not only you, but also helps other people understand what you are going through. Having support from other people who understand is very empowering.

There may be some people in your life who you feel more comfortable asking for practical support rather than the kind of emotional support gained through talking about bladder illness. Some examples of these may be:

- asking a family member to help with more heavy-duty housework
- inviting a friend to an exercise class that teaches pelvic floor muscle training
- having your partner help check where accessible toilets are before a trip.

These hands-on activities may bring about conversations about bladder symptoms, therefore acting as two-fold support. However, if it isn't possible to talk to someone you know, there are many online forums and groups on social media sites where people share their experiences. It's worth checking if the forum or group is moderated however, to make sure that any inappropriate behaviour is controlled.

Sleep problems

Everything feels worse if you can't sleep. As we know, many people with bladder problems don't sleep enough, as often people need to get up in the night to use the bathroom, or they have trouble sleeping due to bladder pain. Sometimes, even when night-time urgency and frequency have diminished with treatment, difficulty sleeping can remain. This is because once we get into a poor sleep habit, our sleep patterns may not automatically snap back into place. To help guide your body back into a good sleep pattern, try these tips:

- Natural light is fundamental to our body's sleep-wake cycle (the circadian rhythm), so try to get outdoors if you can. Even if you can't manage a walk, sitting in the daylight will help to remind your body when it's time for sleep and time to be awake. This will also help boost vitamin D levels.
- Keeping your room dark at night is also important for the brain to recognise it's time for sleep. There are many types of blackout blinds on the market and eye masks that can help with this.
- Noise can stir us from slumber also – if you live in a noisy area, see if white noise helps. The constant sound tends to mask any jarring noises. White noise can be downloaded onto a smartphone, tablet or bought as a noise machine.
- Ensure there is enough air circulating in the room by leaving a window open, even just a crack.
- A cool room is best for sleep – 18°C is the general recommendation.
- Body temperature is also something that can be tweaked for a good sound sleep. It's better to cool down rather than try to warm up your body once in bed – try a warm bath or shower before bed.
- Exercise supports our overall health so don't avoid

movement if you're not sleeping well but schedule your more vigorous activities earlier in the day (definitely not within three or four hours of bedtime).

- Caffeine, cigarettes, alcohol and some medicines can disturb sleep so should be limited or avoided if possible.
- Screens should be kept out of the bedroom, including smartphones, tablets and TVs.

If you've tried all these suggestions and you still can't sleep, or are feeling tired and sleepy in the day, it might be worth trying sleep restriction (see our IBS book), and/or talking to your doctor about sleep problems. She may want to rule out conditions such as sleep apnoea which cause short bouts of wakefulness due to breathing difficulty, or recommend a short course of sleep medication.

Summary and conclusion

We hope that this final chapter has given you some practical ways to deal with the difficulties that bladder problems can cause and also some more general tips to support your health.

A final word

Bladder conditions are common but often hidden, not only from view but from conversation. The symptoms of bladder illness can leave people isolated and unable to enjoy everyday activities and have an impact on relationships. For some of us, urinary issues rob us of our freedom – freedom to travel, socialise and communicate our experience. These problems are similar to other conditions that we have studied over the years, including IBS, IBD and ME/CFS. However, incontinence is not just a part of getting older – there are many things that we as individuals can do to lessen the impact of symptoms on everyday life. These include exercises to improve bladder function, dietary changes to control flare-ups and incontinence products to improve confidence. Medications and medical procedures may also be useful for you so it's worth discussing all options with your doctor.

Talking about symptoms can definitely be the key to the door to better health – during the research for this book we were surprised by how reluctant people were to talk about their bladder problems. In fact, they were much more reluctant than people with other conditions that we have studied. There is still a significant taboo around incontinence, but this can be shattered through exchanging our stories. Knowing you're not the only one with an illness can offer comfort in itself. The ideas and tips from others that we've included may also nudge your recovery onwards. We hope so. We also hope the information in this book guides you to good health because, as Martina states:

I hope my story will be useful and I hope it will help others too.

Martina

We wish you all the best,
Megan and Christine

References

Chapter 1: You are not alone – bladder problems are very common

1. Coyne KS, Sexton CC, Kopp ZS, Ebel-Bitoun C, Milsom I, Chapple C. The impact of overactive bladder on mental health, work productivity and health-related quality of life in the UK and Sweden: results from EpiLUTS. *BJU International* 2011; 108(9): 1459-1471.

2. Milsom I, Abrams P, Cardozo L, Roberts RG, Thüroff J, Wein AJ. How widespread are the symptoms of an overactive bladder and how are they managed? A population-based prevalence study. *BJU International* 2001; 87(9): 760-766.

3. Homma Y, Yamaguchi O, Hayashi K. An epidemiological survey of overactive bladder symptoms in Japan. *BJU International* 2005; 96(9): 1314-1318.

4. Sarici H, Ozgur BC, Telli O, Doluoglu OG, Eroglu M, Bozkurt S. The prevalence of overactive bladder syndrome and urinary incontinence in a Turkish women's population; associated risk factors and effect on quality of life. *Urologia* 2014; 83(2): 93-98.

5. Muller N. What Americans understand and how they are affected by bladder control problems: highlights of recent nationwide consumer research. *Urologic Nursing* 2005; 25(2): 109.

6. Ashley J. Women 'more likely to report ill health than men'. *BBC News*, 26 March 2010. http://news.bbc.co.uk/1/hi/health/8588686.stm

7. Matsumoto S, Hashizume K, Wada N, Hori J, Tamaki G, Kita M, Iwata T, Kakizaki H. Relationship between overactive bladder and

irritable bowel syndrome: a large-scale internet survey in Japan using the overactive bladder symptom score and Rome III criteria. *BJU International* 2013; 111(4): 647-652.

8.   Whorwell PJ, Lupton EW, Erduran D, Wilson K. Bladder smooth muscle dysfunction in patients with irritable bowel syndrome. *Gut* 1986; 27(9): 1014-1017.

9.   Persson R, Wensaas KA, Hanevik K, Eide GE, Langeland N, Rortveit G. The relationship between irritable bowel syndrome, functional dyspepsia, chronic fatigue and overactive bladder syndrome: a controlled study 6 years after acute gastrointestinal infection. *BMC Gastroenterology* 2015; 15(1): 66.

10.   Rubin EB, Buehler AE, Halpern SD. States worse than death among hospitalized patients with serious illnesses. *JAMA Internal Medicine* 2016; 176(10): 1557-1559.

11.   Heyes SM, Harrington A, Bond MJ, Belan I. The lived experiences of people with bladder cancer and their partners: Susan Heyes and colleagues review studies into the effects of bladder cancer diagnosis and treatment on personal relationships. *Cancer Nursing Practice* 2014; 13(9): 25-30.

12.   Bosch PC, Bosch DC. Treating interstitial cystitis/bladder pain syndrome as a chronic disease. *Reviews in Urology* 2014; 16(2): 83.

13.   Li M, Wang L. The Associations of Psychological Stress with Depressive and Anxiety Symptoms among Chinese Bladder and Renal Cancer Patients: The Mediating Role of Resilience. *PloS One* 2016; 11(4): e0154729.

14.   Held PJ, Hanno PM, Wein AJ, Pauly MV, Cahn MA. Epidemiology of interstitial cystitis: 2. In: *Interstitial Cystitis</ita>* London: Springer; 1990: 29-48.

15.   Patel A, Cannon TW, O'Leary M, Xavier M, Erickson J, Leng W, Sweeney D, Chancellor MB, Patel S, Borello-France D. Relationship between overactive bladder (OAB) and sexual activity in women. *Journal of Urology* 2004; 171(4): 90-90.

16.   Webster DC, Brennan T. Use and effectiveness of sexual self-care strategies for interstitial cystitis. *Urologic Nursing* 1995; 15(1): 14-22.

17.   Heidler S, Mert C, Wehrberger C, Temml C, Ponholzer A, Rauchenwald M, Madersbacher S. Impact of overactive bladder symptoms on sexuality in both sexes. *Urologia Internationalis* 2010; 85(4): 443-446.

18. Elstad EA, Taubenberger SP, Botelho EM, Tennstedt SL. Beyond incontinence: the stigma of other urinary symptoms. *Journal of Advanced Nursing* 2010; 66(11): 2460-2470.

19. Koziol JA, Clark DC, Gittes RF, Tan EM. The natural history of interstitial cystitis: a survey of 374 patients. *Journal of Urology* 1993; 149(3): 465-469

20. Troxel WM, Booth M, Buysse DJ, Elliott MN, Suskind AM, Clemens JQ, Berry SH. Sleep disturbances and nocturnal symptoms: relationships with quality of life in a population-based sample of women with interstitial cystitis/bladder pain syndrome. *Journal of Clinical Sleep Medicine* 2014; 10(12): 1331.

21. Newman DK, Koochaki PE. Characteristics and impact of interrupted sleep in women with overactive bladder. *Urologic Nursing* 2011; 31(5): 304.

22. Arroll MA, Dancey CP. *Irritable Bowel Syndrome: navigating your way to recovery.* London: Hammersmith Health Books; 2016.

23. Ginting JV, Tripp DA, Nickel JC, Fitzgerald MP, Mayer R. 2011. Spousal support decreases the negative impact of pain on mental quality of life in women with interstitial cystitis/painful bladder syndrome. *BJU International* 2011; 108(5): 713-717.

Chapter 2: The bladder – what is it and what does it do?

24. El Nahas AM, Bello AK. Chronic kidney disease: the global challenge. *Lancet* 2005; 365(9456): 331-340.

25. Saladin KS, Miller L. *Anatomy & Physiology* London: WCB/McGraw-Hill; 1998.

Chapter 3: How the bladder communicates with the brain

26. Loewy AD, Spyer KM (Eds) *Central Regulation of Autonomic Functions.* Oxford: Oxford University Press; 1990.

27. Swain S, Hughes R, Perry M, Harrison S. Management of lower urinary tract dysfunction in neurological disease: summary of NICE guidance. *BMJ* 2012; 345: e5074.

28. De Sèze M, Ruffion A, Denys P, Joseph PA, Perrouin-Verbe B. The

neurogenic bladder in multiple sclerosis: review of the literature and proposal of management guidelines. *Multiple Sclerosis Journal* 2007; 13(7): 915-928.

29.   Tubaro A, Puccini F, De Nunzio C, Digesu GA, Elneil S, Gobbi C, Khullar V. 2012. The treatment of lower urinary tract symptoms in patients with multiple sclerosis: a systematic review. *Current Urology Reports* 2012; 13(5): 335-342.

30.   Burns AS, Rivas DA, Ditunno JF. The management of neurogenic bladder and sexual dysfunction after spinal cord injury. *Spine* 2001; 26(24S): S129-S136.

31.   Lynch AC, Antony A, Dobbs BR, Frizelle FA. Bowel dysfunction following spinal cord injury. *Spinal Cord* 2001; 39(4): 193.

32.   Park SE, Elliott S, Noonan VK, Thorogood NP, Fallah N, Aludino A, Dvorak MF. Impact of bladder, bowel and sexual dysfunction on health status of people with thoracolumbar spinal cord injuries living in the community. *Journal of Spinal Cord Medicine* 2016; 1-12.

33.   Braaf S, Lennox A, Nunn A, Gabbe B. Social activity and relationship changes experienced by people with bowel and bladder dysfunction following spinal cord injury. *Spinal Cord* 2017; 55(7): 679-686. doi: 10.1038/sc.2017.19.

Chapter 4: Brain gut interactions and microbiota (gut and urinary)

34.   Fernandez-Real JM, Serino M, Blasco G, Puig J, Daunis-i-Estadella J, Ricart W, Burcelin R, Fernández-Aranda F, Portero-Otin M. Gut microbiota interacts with brain microstructure and function. *Journal of Clinical Endocrinology & Metabolism* 2015; 100(12): 4505-4513.

35.   O'Mahony SM, Marchesi JR, Scully P, Codling C, Ceolho AM, Quigley EM, Cryan JF, Dinan TG. Early life stress alters behavior, immunity, and microbiota in rats: implications for irritable bowel syndrome and psychiatric illnesses. *Biological Psychiatry* 2009; 65(3): 263-267.

36.   Galley JD, Nelson MC, Yu Z, Dowd SE, Walter J, Kumar PS, Lyte M, Bailey MT. Exposure to a social stressor disrupts the community structure of the colonic mucosa-associated microbiota. *BMC Microbiology* 2014; 14(1): 189.

37.   Bennet SM, Öhman L, Simrén M. Gut microbiota as potential orchestrators of irritable bowel syndrome. *Gut and Liver* 2015; 9(3): 318.

38. Round JL, Mazmanian SK. The gut microbiome shapes intestinal immune responses during health and disease. *Nature Reviews: Immunology* 2009; 9(5): 313.

39. Nicholson JK, Holmes E, Kinross J, Burcelin R, Gibson G, Jia W, Pettersson S. 2012. Host-gut microbiota metabolic interactions. *Science* 2012; 336(6086): 1262-1267.

40. Goodrich JK, Waters JL, Poole AC, Sutter JL, Koren O, Blekhman R, Beaumont M, Van Treuren W, Knight R, Bell JT, Spector TD. Human genetics shape the gut microbiome. *Cell* 2014; 159(4): 789-799.

41. Palma G, Collins SM, Bercik P, Verdu EF. The microbiota–gut–brain axis in gastrointestinal disorders: stressed bugs, stressed brain or both? *Journal of Physiology* 2014; 592(14): 2989-2997.

42. Luna RA, Foster JA. Gut brain axis: diet microbiota interactions and implications for modulation of anxiety and depression. *Current Opinion in Biotechnology* 2015; 32: 35-41.

43. Nienhouse V, Gao X, Dong Q, Nelson DE, Toh E, McKinley K, Schreckenberger P, Shibata N, Fok CS, Mueller ER, Brubaker L. Interplay between bladder microbiota and urinary antimicrobial peptides: mechanisms for human urinary tract infection risk and symptom severity. *PLoS One* 2014; 9(12): e114185.

44. Brubaker L, Wolfe A. The urinary microbiota: a paradigm shift for bladder disorders?. *Current Opinion in Obstetrics and Gynecology* 2016; 28(5):407-412.

45. Shoskes DA, Altemus J, Polackwich AS, Tucky B, Wang H, Eng C. The urinary microbiome differs significantly between patients with chronic prostatitis / chronic pelvic pain syndrome and controls as well as between patients with different clinical phenotypes. *Urology* 2016; 92: 26-32.

46. Karstens L, Asquith M, Davin S, Stauffer P, Fair D, Gregory WT, Rosenbaum JT, McWeeney SK, Nardos R. Does the urinary microbiome play a role in urgency urinary incontinence and its severity?. *Frontiers in Cellular and Infection Microbiology* 2016; 6.

Chapter 5: Urinary incontinence, overactivity and retention

47. Elenskaia K, Haidvogel K, Heidinger C, Doerfler D, Umek W, Hanzal E. The greatest taboo: urinary incontinence as a source of

shame and embarrassment. *Wiener Klinische Wochenschrift* 2011; 123(19): 607-610.

48. Horrocks S, Somerset M, Stoddart H, Peters TJ. What prevents older people from seeking treatment for urinary incontinence? A qualitative exploration of barriers to the use of community continence services. *Family Practice* 2004; 21(6): 689-696.

49. Haylen BT, De Ridder D, Freeman RM, Swift SE, Berghmans B, Lee J, Monga A, Petri E, Rizk DE, Sand PK, Schaer GN. An International Urogynecological Association (IUGA)/International Continence Society (ICS) joint report on the terminology for female pelvic floor dysfunction. *International Urogynecology Journal* 2010; 21(1): 5-26.

50. Sangsawang B, Sangsawang N. Stress urinary incontinence in pregnant women: a review of prevalence, pathophysiology, and treatment. *International Urogynecology Journal* 2013; 24(6): 901-912.

51. Chaliha C, Kalia V, Stanton SL, Monga ASH, Sultan AH. Antenatal prediction of postpartum urinary and fecal incontinence. *Obstetrics & Gynecology* 1999; 94(5): 689-694.

52. Van Geelen JM, Lemmens WAJG, Eskes TKAB, Martin CB. The urethral pressure profile in pregnancy and after delivery in healthy nulliparous women. *American Journal of Obstetrics and Gynecology* 1982; 144(6): 636-649.

53. Falconer C, Ekman G, Malmstrom A, Ulmsten U. Decreased collagen synthesis in stress-incontinent women. *Obstetrics & Gynecology* 1994; 84(4, Part 1): 583-586.

54. Smith MD, Hussain M, Seth JH, Kazkaz H, Panicker JN. Stress urinary incontinence as the presenting complaint of benign joint hypermobility syndrome. *Journal of the Royal Society of Medicine: Short Reports* 2012; 3(9): 66.

55. Jura YH, Townsend MK, Curhan GC, Resnick NM, Grodstein F. Caffeine intake, and the risk of stress, urgency and mixed urinary incontinence. *Journal of Urology* 2011; 185(5): 1775-1780.

56. Bryant CM, Douvell CJ, Fairbrother G. Caffeine reduction education to improve urinary symptoms. *British Journal of Nursing* 2002; 11(8): 8.

57. Pons ME, Clota MP. Coital urinary incontinence: impact on quality of life as measured by the King's Health Questionnaire. *International Urogynecology Journal* 2008; 19(5): 621-625.

58. Kim YH, Seo JT, Yoon H. The effect of overactive bladder syndrome on the sexual quality of life in Korean young and

middle aged women. *International Journal of Impotence Research* 2005; 17(2): 158-163.

59.   Temml C, Heidler S, Ponholzer A, Madersbacher S. Prevalence of the overactive bladder syndrome by applying the International Continence Society definition. *European Urology* 2005; 48(4): 622-627.

60.   Milsom I, Abrams P, Cardozo L, Roberts RG, Thüroff J, Wein AJ. How widespread are the symptoms of an overactive bladder and how are they managed? A population-based prevalence study. *BJU International* 2001; 87(9): 760-766.

61.   Abrams P, Cardozo L, Fall M, Griffiths D, Rosier P, Ulmsten U, van Kerrebroeck P, Victor A, Wein A. The standardisation of terminology of lower urinary tract function: report from the Standardisation Sub-committee of the International Continence Society. *American Journal of Obstetrics and Gynecology* 2002; 1(187): 116-126.

62.   Daneshgari F, Liu G, Birder L, Hanna-Mitchell AT, Chacko S. Diabetic bladder dysfunction: current translational knowledge. *Journal of Urology* 2009; 182(6): S18-S26.

63.   Lamonerie L, Marret E, Deleuze A, Lembert N, Dupont M, Bonnet F. Prevalence of postoperative bladder distension and urinary retention detected by ultrasound measurement. *British Journal of Anaesthesia* 2004; 92(4): 544-546.

Chapter 6: Cystitis and interstitial cystitis

64.   Foxman B. The epidemiology of urinary tract infection. *Nat Rev Urol* 2010; 7: 653–660.

64A.   Boucher HW. Challenges in anti-infective development in the era of bad bugs, no drugs: a regulatory perspective using the example of bloodstream infection as an indication. *Clinical Infectious Diseases* 2010; 50 (Supplement 1): S4-S9.

64B.   Jepson RG, Williams G, Craig G. Cochrane Review: Cranberries for preventing urinary tract infections. *Cochrane Database of Systematic Reviews* 10; 17 October 2012. (www.cochrane.org/ CD001321/RENAL_cranberries-for-preventing-urinary-tract-infections accessed 6 November 2017)

65.   MacDiarmid SA, Sand PK. Diagnosis of interstitial cystitis/painful bladder syndrome in patients with overactive bladder symptoms. *Reviews in Urology* 2007; 9(1): 9.

66. Parsons CL, Dell J, Stanford EJ, Bullen M, Kahn BS, Waxell T, Koziol JA. 2002. Increased prevalence of interstitial cystitis: previously unrecognized urologic and gynecologic cases identified using a new symptom questionnaire and intravesical potassium sensitivity. *Urology* 2002; 60(4): 573-578.

67. Urb M. Sheppard DC. The role of mast cells in the defence against pathogens. *PLoS Pathology* 2012; 8(4): e1002619.

68. Gamper M, Regauer S, Welter J, Eberhard J, Viereck V. Are mast cells still good biomarkers for bladder pain syndrome/interstitial cystitis?. *Journal of Urology* 2015; 193(6): 1994-2000.

69. Parsons CL. The role of the urinary epithelium in the pathogenesis of interstitial cystitis/prostatitis/urethritis. *Urology* 2007; 69(4): S9-S16.

70. Parsons CL, Shaw T, Berecz Z, Su Y, Zupkas P, Argade S. Role of urinary cations in the aetiology of bladder symptoms and interstitial cystitis. *BJU International* 2014; 114(2): 286-293.

71. Arroll MA, Dancey CP. *Irritable Bowel Syndrome: navigating your way to recovery.* London: Hammersmith Health Books; 2016.

72. Hohenfellner M, Nunes L, Schmidt RA, Lampel A, Thüroff JW, Tanagho EA. Interstitial cystitis: increased sympathetic innervation and related neuropeptide synthesis. *Journal of Urology* 1992; 147(3): 587-591.

73. Peters KM, Carrico DJ, Kalinowski SE, Ibrahim IA, Diokno AC. 2007. Prevalence of pelvic floor dysfunction in patients with interstitial cystitis. *Urology* 2007; 70(1): 16-18.

74. Van De Merwe JP, Yamada T, Sakamoto Y. 2003. Systemic aspects of interstitial cystitis, immunology and linkage with autoimmune disorders. *International Journal of Urology* 2003; 10(s1): S35-S38.

75. Davis NF, Brady CM, Creagh T. Interstitial cystitis/painful bladder syndrome: epidemiology, pathophysiology and evidence-based treatment options. *European Journal of Obstetrics & Gynecology and Reproductive Biology* 2014; 175: 30-37.

76. Warren JW, Keay SK, Meyers D, Xu J. Concordance of interstitial cystitis in monozygotic and dizygotic twin pairs. *Urology* 2001; 57(6): 22-25.

77. Chung MK, Chung RP, Gordon D. 2005. Interstitial cystitis and endometriosis in patients with chronic pelvic pain: the "evil twins" syndrome. *JSLS* 2005; 9(1): 25-29.

78. Sant GR, Hanno PM. 2001. Interstitial cystitis: current issues and controversies in diagnosis. *Urology* 2001; 57(6): 82-88.

Chapter 7: Bladder cancer

79. Sharma S, Ksheersagar P, Sharma P. Diagnosis and treatment of bladder cancer. *American Family Physician* 2009; 80(7): 717-23.

80. Pashos CL, Botteman MF, Laskin BL, Redaelli A. Bladder cancer. *Cancer Practice* 2002; 10(6): 311-322.

81. www.ons.gov.uk/peoplepopulationandcommunity/ healthandsocialcare/conditionsanddiseases/bulletins/ cancerregistrationstatisticsengland/previousReleases

82. Jankovic S, Radosavljevic V. Risk factors for bladder cancer. *Tumori* 2007; 93(1): 4.

83. Kirkali Z, Chan T, Manoharan M, et al. Bladder cancer: epidemiology, staging and grading, and diagnosis. *Urology* 2005; 66(6 suppl 1): 4-34.

84. Vineis P, Simonato L. Proportion of lung and bladder cancers in males resulting from occupation: a systematic approach. *Archives of Environmental Health* 1991; 46(1): 6-15.

85. Gago-Dominguez M, Castelao JE, Yuan JM, Yu MC, Ross RK. Use of permanent hair dyes and bladder-cancer risk. *International Journal of Cancer* 2001; 91(4): 575-579.

86. Kogevinas, M, Fernandez F, Garcia-Closas M, Tardon A, Garcia-Closas R, Serra C, Carrato A, Castano-Vinyals G, Yeager M, Chanock SJ, Lloreta J. Hair dye use is not associated with risk for bladder cancer: evidence from a case-control study in Spain. *European Journal of Cancer* 2006; 42(10): 1448-1454

87. Wyszynski A, Tanyos SA, Rees JR, Marsit CJ, Kelsey KT, Schned AR, Pendleton EM, Celaya MO, Zens MS, Karagas MR, Andrew AS. Body mass and smoking are modifiable risk factors for recurrent bladder cancer. *Cancer* 2014; 120(3): 408-414.

88. Honma I, Masumori N, Sato E, et al. Local recurrence after radical cystectomy for invasive bladder cancer: an analysis of predictive factors. *Urology* 2004; 64: 744-748.

89. Sun JW, Zhao LG, Yang Y, Ma X, Wang YY, Xiang YB. Obesity and risk of bladder cancer: a dose-response meta-analysis of 15 cohort studies. *PloS One* 2015; 10(3): e0119313.

90. Shephard RJ. Physical activity in the prevention and management of bladder cancer. *Journal of Sports Medicine and Physical Fitness* 2017; 57(10):1359-1366. doi: 10.23736/S0022-4707.17.06830-X.

91. Karvinen KH, Courneya KS, North S, Venner P. Associations between exercise and quality of life in bladder cancer survivors: a population-based study. *Cancer Epidemiology and Prevention Biomarkers* 2007; 16(5): 984-990.

92. Chu H, Wang M, Zhang Z. Bladder cancer epidemiology and genetic susceptibility. *J Biomed Res* 2013; 27(3): 170-178.

93. Larsson SC, Orsini N, Brismar K, Wolk A. Diabetes mellitus and risk of bladder cancer: a meta-analysis. *Diabetologia* 2006; 49(12): 2819-2823.

94. Dormandy JA, Charbonnel B, Eckland DJ, Erdmann E, Massi-Benedetti M, Moules IK, Skene AM, Tan MH, Lefèbvre PJ, Murray GD, Standl E. 2005. Secondary prevention of macrovascular events in patients with type 2 diabetes in the PROactive Study (PROspective pioglitAzone Clinical Trial In macroVascular Events): a randomised controlled trial. *Lancet* 2005; 366(9493): 1279-1289.

95. Groah SL, Weitzenkamp DA, Lammertse DP, Whiteneck GG, Lezotte DC, Hamman RF. Excess risk of bladder cancer in spinal cord injury: evidence for an association between indwelling catheter use and bladder cancer. *Archives of Physical Medicine and Rehabilitation* 2002; 83(3): 346-351.

96. Pedotti P, Cardillo M, Rossini G, Arcuri V, et al. 2003. Incidence of cancer after kidney transplant: results from the North Italy transplant program. *Transplantation* 2003; 76(10): 1448-1451.

97. Gutierrez-Dalmau A, Campistol JM. Immunosuppressive therapy and malignancy in organ transplant recipients. *Drugs* 2007; 67(8): 1167-1198.

98. Bourrier A, Carrat F, Colombel JF, Bouvier AM, Abitbol V, Marteau P, Cosnes J, Simon T, Peyrin-Biroulet L, Beaugerie L. Excess risk of urinary tract cancers in patients receiving thiopurines for inflammatory bowel disease: a prospective observational cohort study. *Alimentary Pharmacology & Therapeutics* 2016; 43(2): 252-261.

99. Abol-Enein H. Infection: is it a cause of bladder cancer?. *Scandinavian Journal of Urology and Nephrology* 2008; 42(sup 218): 79-84.

100. Michaud DS, Platz EA, Giovannucci E. Gonorrhoea and male bladder cancer in a prospective study. *British Journal of Cancer* 2007; 96(1): 169-171.

101. Foley KL, Farmer DF, Petronis VM, Smith RG, McGraw S, Smith K, Carver CS, Avis N. 2006. A qualitative exploration of the cancer experience among long-term survivors: comparisons by cancer type, ethnicity, gender, and age. *Psycho-Oncology* 2006; 15(3): 248-258.

Chapter 8: Medical investigations

102. Clemens JQ, Calhoun EA, Litwin MS, et al. A survey of primary care physician practices in the diagnosis and management of women with interstitial cystitis/painful bladder syndrome. *Urology* 2010;76:323-8. http://dx.doi.org/10.1016/j.urology.2009.12.047

103. www.guysandstthomas.nhs.uk/resources/patient-information/gynaecology/Bladder-diary.pdf

Chapter 9: Behavioural treatments

104. Burgio KL. Current perspectives on management of urgency using bladder and behavioral training. *Journal of the American Academy of Nurse Practitioners* 2004; 16(10 Suppl): 4-7.

105. Lee HE, Cho SY, Lee S, Kim M, Oh SJ. 2013. Short-term effects of a systematized bladder training program for idiopathic overactive bladder: a prospective study. *International Neurology Journal* 2013; 17(1): 11.

106. Miller E. Why I wrote a comedy show about incontinence. *The Guardian* 10 August 2017. https://amp.theguardian.com/healthcare-network/2017/aug/10/why-wrote-comedy-show-incontinence-edinburgh-fringe (Accessed 1 December 2017)

107. Boyle R, Hay-Smith EJ, Cody JD, Mørkved S. 2012. Pelvic floor muscle training for prevention and treatment of urinary and faecal incontinence in antenatal and postnatal women. *Cochrane Database Systematic Reviews* 2012; 10.

108. Cavkaytar S, Kokanali MK, Topcu HO, Aksakal OS, Doğanay M. Effect of home-based Kegel exercises on quality of life in women with stress and mixed urinary incontinence. *Journal of Obstetrics and Gynaecology* 2015; 35(4): 407-410.

Chapter 10: Food and drink

109. Jura YH, Townsend MK, Curhan GC, Resnick NM, Grodstein F. 2011. Caffeine intake and risk of stress, urgency, and mixed urinary incontinence. *Journal of Urology* 2011; 185(5): 1775–1780. doi.org/10.1016/j.juro.2011.01.003

110. Dallosso HM, Matthews RJ, McGrother CW, Donaldson MM,

Shaw C. The association of diet and other lifestyle factors with the onset of overactive bladder: a longitudinal study in men. *Public Health Nutrition* 2004; 7(7): 885-891.

111. Zeevi D, Korem T, Zmora N, Israeli D, Rothschild D, Weinberger A, Ben-Yacov O, Lador D, Avnit-Sagi T, Lotan-Pompan M, Suez J. Personalized nutrition by prediction of glycemic responses. *Cell* 2015; 163(5): 1079-1094.

112. Cryan JF, Dinan TG. Mind-altering microorganisms: the impact of the gut microbiota on brain and behaviour. *Nature Reviews: Neuroscience* 2012; 13(10): 701-712.

113. Martin FPJ, Rezzi S, Peré-Trepat E, Kamlage B, Collino S, Leibold E, Kastler J, Rein D, Fay LB, Kochhar S. 2009. Metabolic effects of dark chocolate consumption on energy, gut microbiota, and stress-related metabolism in free-living subjects. *Journal of Proteome Research* 2009; 8(12): 5568-5579.

114. Parvez S, Malik KA, Ah Kang S, Kim HY. 2006. Probiotics and their fermented food products are beneficial for health. *Journal of Applied Microbiology* 2006; 100(6): 1171-1185.

115. Elmer GW. 2001. Probiotics: "living drugs". *American Journal of Health System Pharmacy* 2001; 58(12): 1101-1109.

116. Reid G, Bruce AW. Selection of Lactobacillus strains for urogenital probiotic applications. *Journal of Infectious Diseases* 2001; 183(Supplement 1): S77-S80.

117. Stapleton AE, Au-Yeung M, Hooton TM, Fredricks DN, Roberts PL, Czaja CA, Yarova-Yarovaya Y, Fiedler T, Cox M, Stamm WE. Randomized, placebo-controlled phase 2 trial of a Lactobacillus crispatus probiotic given intravaginally for prevention of recurrent urinary tract infection. *Clinical Infectious Diseases* 2011; 52(10): 1212-1217.

118. Ueda T, Yoshida T, Tanoue H, Ito M, Tamaki M, Ito Y, Yoshimura N. Urine alkalization improves the problems of pain and sleep in hypersensitive bladder syndrome. *International Journal of Urology* 2014; 21(5): 512-517.

119. Demirbas A, Sarici H, Kilinc MF, Telli O, Ozgur BC, Doluoglu OG, Bozkurt S. The relationship between acidic urinary pH and overactive bladder; alkalization of urine improves the symptoms of overactive bladder. *Urologia Internationalis* 2015; 95(2): 223-226.

Chapter 11: Lifestyle changes

120. EFSA Panel on Dietetic Products, Nutrition, and Allergies. Scientific opinion on dietary reference values for water. *EFSA Journal* 2010; 8(3):1459.

121. Nickel JC, Tripp DA, Pontari M, Moldwin R, Mayer R, Carr LK, Doggweiler R, Yang CC, Mishra N, Nordling J. 2010. Psychosocial phenotyping in women with interstitial cystitis/painful bladder syndrome: a case control study. *Journal of Urology* 2010; 183(1): 167-172.

122. Knight S, Luft J, Nakagawa S, Katzman WB. 2012. Comparisons of pelvic floor muscle performance, anxiety, quality of life and life stress in women with dry overactive bladder compared with asymptomatic women. *BJU International* 2012; 109(11): 1685-1689.

123. Coyne KS, Wein AJ, Tubaro A, Sexton CC, Thompson CL, Kopp ZS, Aiyer LP. The burden of lower urinary tract symptoms: evaluating the effect of LUTS on health-related quality of life, anxiety and depression: EpiLUTS. *BJU International* 2009; 103(s3): 4-11.

124. Al-Zalabani, A.H., Stewart, K.F., Wesselius, A., Schols, A.M. and Zeegers, M.P., 2016. Modifiable risk factors for the prevention of bladder cancer: a systematic review of meta-analyses. *European journal of epidemiology*, 31(9), pp.811-851.

125. Ferkol, T. and Schraufnagel, D., 2014. The global burden of respiratory disease. *Annals of the American Thoracic Society*, 11(3), pp.404-406.

126. Chang, S.J., Chiang, I.N., Lin, C.D., Hsieh, C.H. and Yang, S.S.D., 2015. Obese children at higher risk for having overactive bladder symptoms: A community-based study. *Neurourology and urodynamics*, 34(2), pp.123-127.

127. Ramalingam, K. and Monga, A., 2015. Obesity and pelvic floor dysfunction. *Best practice & research Clinical obstetrics & gynaecology*, 29(4), pp.541-547.

128. Subak, L.L., Wing, R., West, D.S., Franklin, F., Vittinghoff, E., Creasman, J.M., Richter, H.E., Myers, D., Burgio, K.L., Gorin, A.A. and Macer, J., 2009. Weight loss to treat urinary incontinence in overweight and obese women. *New England Journal of Medicine*, 360(5), pp.481-490.

129. Mosley M, Spencer M. *The Fast Diet-Revised & Updated: Lose Weight,*

Stay Healthy, and Live Longer with the Simple Secret of Intermittent Fasting. London: Simon and Schuster; 2015.

130. Varady KA. Intermittent versus daily calorie restriction: which diet regimen is more effective for weight loss? *Obesity Reviews* 2011; 12(7).

131. Geliebter A, Aversa A. Emotional eating in overweight, normal weight, and underweight individuals. *Eating Behaviors* 2003; 3(4): 341-347.

132. Maeda T, Tomita M, Nakazawa A, Sakai G, Funakoshi S, Komatsuda A, Ito Y, Nagata H, Tsukada N, Nakamura S. 2017. Female Functional Constipation Is Associated with Overactive Bladder Symptoms and Urinary Incontinence. *BioMed Research International* 2017. doi: 10.1155/2017/2138073

133. Benner JS, Nichol MB, Rovner ES, Jumadilova Z, Alvir J, Hussein M, Fanning K, Trocio JN, Brubaker L. Patient-reported reasons for discontinuing overactive bladder medication. *BJU International* 2010; 105(9): 1276-1282.

134. Arnaud MJ. Mild dehydration: a risk factor of constipation? *European Journal of Clinical Nutrition* 2003; 57: S88-S95.

135. Bi L, Triadafilopoulos G. Exercise and gastrointestinal function and disease: an evidence-based review of risks and benefits. *Clinical Gastroenterology and Hepatology* 2003; 1(5): 345-355.

136. De Schryver AM, Keulemans YC, Peters HP, Akkermans LM, Smout AJ, De Vries WR, Van Berge-Henegouwen GP. 2005. Effects of regular physical activity on defecation pattern in middle-aged patients complaining of chronic constipation. *Scandinavian Journal of Gastroenterology* 2005; 40(4): 422-429.

137. Jakicic JM, Marcus BH, Gallagher KI, Napolitano M, Lang W. 2003. Effect of exercise duration and intensity on weight loss in overweight, sedentary women: a randomized trial. *JAMA* 2003; 290(10): 1323-1330.

Chapter 12: Medications for bladder conditions

138. Andersson KE. New developments in the management of overactive bladder: focus on mirabegron and onabotulinumtoxinA. *Ther Clin Risk Manag* 2013; 9(9): 161-70.

139. Chapple CR, Khullar V, Gabriel Z, Muston D, Bitoun CE, Weinstein D. 2008. The effects of antimuscarinic treatments in

overactive bladder: an update of a systematic review and meta-analysis. *European Urology* 2008; 54(3): 543-562.

140. Van Kerrebroeck P, Kreder K, Jonas U, Zinner N, Wein A, Tolterodine Study Group. Tolterodine once-daily: superior efficacy and tolerability in the treatment of the overactive bladder. *Urology* 2001; 57(3): 414-421.

141. Chapple CR, Cardozo L, Nitti VW, Siddiqui E, Michel MC. Mirabegron in overactive bladder: a review of efficacy, safety, and tolerability. *Neurourology and Urodynamics* 2014; 33(1): 17-30.

142. Nitti VW, Chapple CR, Walters C, Blauwet MB, Herschorn S, Milsom I, Auerbach S, Radziszewski P. 2014. Safety and tolerability of the ☐3☐adrenoceptor agonist mirabegron, for the treatment of overactive bladder: results of a prospective pooled analysis of three 12-week randomised Phase III trials and of a 1-year randomised Phase III trial. *International Journal of Clinical Practice* 2014; 68(8): 972-985.

143. Chapple C, Patel A. Botulinum toxin—new mechanisms, new therapeutic directions? *European Urology* 2006; 49(4): 606-608.

144. Karsenty G, Denys P, Amarenco G, De Seze M, Gamé X, Haab F, Kerdraon J, Perrouin-Verbe B, Ruffion A, Saussine C, Soler JM. Botulinum toxin A (Botox®) intradetrusor injections in adults with neurogenic detrusor overactivity/neurogenic overactive bladder: a systematic literature review. *European Urology* 2008; 53(2): 275-287.

145. Akiyama Y, Nomiya A, Niimi A, Yamada Y, Fujimura T, Nakagawa T, Fukuhara H, Kume H, Igawa Y, Homma Y. Botulinum toxin type A injection for refractory interstitial cystitis: A randomized comparative study and predictors of treatment response. *International Journal of Urology* 2015; 22(9): 835-841.

146. Anger JT, Weinberg A, Suttorp MJ, Litwin MS, Shekelle PG. 2010. Outcomes of intravesical botulinum toxin for idiopathic overactive bladder symptoms: a systematic review of the literature. *The Journal of Urology* 2010; 183(6): 2258-2264.

147. Millard RJ, Moore K, Rencken R, Yalcin I, Bump RC. 2004. Duloxetine vs placebo in the treatment of stress urinary incontinence: a four-continent randomized clinical trial. *BJU International* 2004; 93(3): 311-318.

148. Davis EL, El Khoudary SR, Talbott EO, Davis J, Regan LJ. Safety and efficacy of the use of intravesical and oral pentosan

polysulfate sodium for interstitial cystitis: a randomized double-blind clinical trial. *Journal of Urology?*ital> 2008; 179(1): 177-185

149. Parsons CL. 2005. Successful downregulation of bladder sensory nerves with combination of heparin and alkalinized lidocaine in patients with interstitial cystitis. *Urology* 2005; 65(1): 45-48.

Chapter 13: Other medical devices and surgery

150. Roumeguère T, Quackels TH, Bollens R, De Groote A, Zlotta A, Bossche MV, Schulman C. 2005. Trans-obturator vaginal tape (TOT®) for female stress incontinence: one year follow-up in 120 patients. *European Urology* 2005; 48(5): 805-809.

151. Nilsson CG, Palva K, Rezapour M, Falconer C. Eleven years prospective follow-up of the tension-free vaginal tape procedure for treatment of stress urinary incontinence. *International Urogynecology Journal* 2008; 19(8): 1043-1047.

152. Lapitan MC, Cody JD, Grant A. 2009. Open retropubic colposuspension for urinary incontinence in women. *Cochrane Database Systematic Reviews* 2009; 4.

153. Eriksen BC, Hagen B, Eik-Nes SH, Molne K, Mjølnererd OK, Romslo L. Long-term effectiveness of the Burch colposuspension in female urinary stress incontinence. *Acta Obstetricia et Gynecologica Scandinavica* 1990; 69(1): 45-50.

154. Van der Aa F, Drake MJ, Kasyan GR, Petrolekas A, Cornu JN, Young Academic Urologists Functional Urology Group. The artificial urinary sphincter after a quarter of a century: a critical systematic review of its use in male non-neurogenic incontinence. *European Urology* 2013; 63(4): 681-689.

155. Greenwell TJ, Venn SN, Mundy AR. Augmentation cystoplasty. *BJU International* 2001; 88(6): 511-525.

156. McGuire MS, Grimaldi G, Grotas J, Russo P. The type of urinary diversion after radical cystectomy significantly impacts on the patient's quality of life. *Annals of Surgical Oncology* 2000; 7(1): 4-8.

157. Lightner DJ. Review of the available urethral bulking agents. *Current Opinion in Urology* 2002; 12(4): 333-338.

158. Kerr LA. Bulking agents in the treatment of stress urinary incontinence: history, outcomes, patient populations, and reimbursement profile. *Reviews in Urology* 2005; 7(Suppl 1): pS3.

159. Siegel SW, Catanzaro F, Dijkema HE, Elhilali MM, Fowler
CJ, Gajewski JB, Hassouna MM, Janknegt RA, Jonas U, van
Kerrebroeck PE, a Nijeholt AL. 2000. Long-term results of a
multicenter study on sacral nerve stimulation for treatment of
urinary urge incontinence, urgency-frequency, and retention.
Urology 2000; 56(6): 87-91.

160. Peters KM, MacDiarmid SA, Wooldridge LS, Leong FC, Shobeiri
SA, Rovner ES, Siegel SW, Tate SB, Jarnagin BK, Rosenblatt
PL, Feagins BA. Randomized trial of percutaneous tibial nerve
stimulation versus extended-release tolterodine: results from the
overactive bladder innovative therapy trial. *Journal of Urology* 2009;
182(3): 1055-1061.

161. MacDiarmid SA, Peters KM, Shobeiri SA, Wooldridge LS,
Rovner ES, Leong FC, Siegel SW, Tate SB, Feagins BA. Long-
term durability of percutaneous tibial nerve stimulation for the
treatment of overactive bladder. *Journal of Urology* 2010; 183(1):
234-240.

162. Brazzelli M, Murray A, Fraser C. 2006. Efficacy and safety of sacral
nerve stimulation for urinary urge incontinence: a systematic
review. *Journal of Urology* 2006; 175(3): 835-841.

Chapter 14: Complementary and alternative medicine (CAM)

163. Philippou Y, Hadjipavlou M, Khan S, Rane A. Complementary and
alternative medicine (CAM) in prostate and bladder cancer. *BJU
International* 2013; 112(8): 1073-1079.

164. Barnes PM, Powell-Griner E, McFann K, Nahin RL.
Complementary and alternative medicine use among adults:
United States, 2002. *Seminars in Integrative Medicine* 2004; 2(2):
54-71.

165. Arroll MA, Dancey CP. *Invisible Illness: Coping with Misunderstood
Conditions*. London: SPCK; 2014.

166. Robinson NG. 2012. One Medicine, One Acupuncture. *Animals*
2012; 2(3): 395-414.

167. Graham P, Cook T. Acupuncture for the treatment of overactive
bladder. *Journal of the Association of Chartered Physiotherapists in
Women's Health* 2008; 102: 53-58

168. Yuan Z, He C, Yan S, Huang D, Wang H, Tang W. 2015. Acupuncture for overactive bladder in female adult: a randomized controlled trial. *World Journal of Urology* 2015; 33(9): 1303-1308.

169. Alraek T, Baerheim A. 'An empty and happy feeling in the bladder…': health changes experienced by women after acupuncture for recurrent cystitis. *Complementary Therapies in Medicine* 2001; 9(4): 219-223.

170. Honjo H, Kawauchi A, Ukimura O, Soh J, Mizutani Y, Miki T. 2002. Treatment of monosymptomatic nocturnal enuresis by acupuncture: A preliminary study. *International Journal of Urology* 2002; 9(12): 672-676.

171. Miller V, Carruthers HR, Morris J, Hasan SS, Archbold S, Whorwell PJ. Hypnotherapy for irritable bowel syndrome: an audit of one thousand adult patients. *Alimentary Pharmacology & Therapeutics* 2015; 41(9): 844-855.

172. Economakis TB. Just in case: Gaining a sense of control over detrusor instability through hypnotherapy. *Australian Journal of Clinical and Experimental Hypnosis* 2007; 35(1): 54-62.

173. Cao Y, Cao R, Bråkenhielm E. 2002. Antiangiogenic mechanisms of diet-derived polyphenols. *Journal of Nutritional Biochemistry* 2002; 13(7): 380-390.

174. Kajiwara M, Mutaguchi K. 2008. Clinical efficacy and tolerability of gosha-jinki-gan, Japanese traditional herbal medicine, in females with overactive bladder. *Acta Urol Jpn* 2008; 54(2): 95-99.

175. Emineke S, Cooper AJ, Fouch S, Birch BR, Lwaleed BA. Diluted honey inhibits biofilm formation: potential application in urinary catheter management? *Journal of Clinical Pathology* 2017; 70(2):140-144. doi: 10.1136/jclinpath-2015-203546.

176. Ishaq F, Malhotra D, Khan A. Antioxidant and antimicrobial activity of pomegranate (punica gratanum) extract against urinary tract infections (uti) pathogens. *Pharma Science Monitor* 2013; 4(3): 355-368.

177. Nishimura M, Ohkawara T, Sato H, Takeda H, Nishihira J. Pumpkin seed oil extracted from Cucurbita maxima improves urinary disorder in human overactive bladder. *Journal of Traditional and Complementary Medicine* 2014; 4(1): 72-74.

178. Katske F, Shoskes DA, Sender M, Poliakin R, Gagliano K, Rajfer J. Treatment of interstitial cystitis with a quercetin supplement.

Techniques in Urology 2001; 7(1): 44-46.

179.   Amaral AF, Cantor KP, Silverman DT, Malats N. Selenium
       and bladder cancer risk: a meta-analysis. *Cancer Epidemiology
       Biomarkers & Prevention* 2010; 19(9), 2407-2415.

180.   Hertting O, Holm Å, Lüthje P, Brauner H, Dyrdak R, Jonasson AF,
       Wiklund P, Chromek M, Brauner A. 2010. Vitamin D induction
       of the human antimicrobial peptide cathelicidin in the urinary
       bladder. *PLoS One* 2010; 5(12): e15580.

Chapter 15: Additional tips on coping with bladder conditions

181.   Carrico DJ, Peters KM, Diokno AC. Guided imagery for women
       with interstitial cystitis: results of a prospective, randomized
       controlled pilot study. *Journal of Alternative and Complementary
       Medicine* 2008; 14(1): 53-60.

182.   Waetjen LE, Liao S, Johnson WO, Sampselle CM, Sternfield B,
       Harlow SD, Gold EB. Study of Women's Health Across the Nation,
       2006. Factors associated with prevalent and incident urinary
       incontinence in a cohort of midlife women: a longitudinal analysis
       of data: study of women's health across the nation. *American
       Journal of Epidemiology* 2007; 165(3): 309-318.

Appendix 1: Useful addresses

General

Bladder Health UK
Kings Court
17 School Road
Birmingham B28 8JG
Tel: 0121 702 0820
Email: General enquiries: info@bladderhealthuk.org
Membership enquiries: susannah@bladderhealthuk.org
Business enquiries: suzanne@bladderhealthuk.org
Website: http://bladderhealthuk.org/

Bladder & Bowel Community
7 The Court
Holywell Business Park
Northfield Road
Southam CV47 0FS
Telephone general enquiries: 01926 357220
Email: help@bladderandbowel.org
Medical helpline: 0800 031 5412

OAB Outlook (Ireland)
Website: www.oab.ie

Bladder cancer

Action Bladder Cancer UK (ABC UK)
6 Trull Farm Buildings
Tetbury
Gloucestershire GL8 8SQ
Tel: 0300 302 0085
Fax: 01285 841 576
E-mail: info@actionbladdercanceruk.org
Website: http://actionbladdercanceruk.org/

Cancer Research UK
PO BOX 1561
Oxford OX4 9GZ
Tel: 0300 123 1022
To speak to a nurse: 0808 800 4040
Fax: 020 3469 6400
Email via the website
Website: www.cancerresearchuk.org

Macmillan Cancer Support
Head office: 020 7840 7840
Support line: 0808 808 00 00 (Monday-Friday, 9:00 am to 8:00 pm)
Online contact form: www.macmillan.org.uk/about-us/contact-us/ask-macmillan-form.html
Website: www.macmillan.org.uk/

Irish Cancer Society
Cancer Nurseline: 1 800 200 700 (freefone in Republic of Ireland)
Website: www.cancer.ie/cancer-information/bladder-cancer

Disability services

Government portal with information about disability rights and support in the UK
Website: www.gov.uk/browse/disabilities

National Key Scheme – Disability Rights UK
CAN Mezzanine
East Road
London N1 6AH
Tel: 020 7250 8191
Disabled Access: Yes
Email: sales@disabilityrightsuk.org
Website: www.disabilityrightsuk.org/

Complementary and alternative medicine

The British Acupuncture Council
63 Jeddo Road
London W12 9HQ
Tel: 020 8735 0400
Fax: 020 8735 0404
Online contact form: www.acupuncture.org.uk/The-British-Acupuncture-Council.html
Website: www.acupuncture.org.uk/

The Hypnotherapy Association UK
14 Crown Street
Chorley
Lancashire PR7 1DX
Tel: 01257 262124
Email: b.h.a@btconnect.com
Website: www.thehypnotherapyassociation.co.uk

The National Hypnotherapy Society
PO Box 131
Arundel
West Sussex BN18 8BR UK
Tel: 0870 850 3387
Email: admin@nationalhypnotherapysociety.org
Website: www.nationalhypnotherapysociety.org

The General Hypnotherapy Standards Council (GHSC) and General Hypnotherapy Register (GHR)
PO Box 204
Lymington SO41 6WP
Email: admin@general-hypnotherapy-register.com
Website: www.general-hypnotherapy-register.com

Complementary and Natural Healthcare Council
83 Victoria Street
London SW1H 0HW
Tel: 020 3178 2199 (Monday to Friday, 9.30 am-5.30 pm)
Email: info@cnhc.org.uk
Website: www.cnhc.org.uk

Appendix 2: Top 10 tips for a healthy bladder

As prevention is always better than cure, we finish with these pointers to keeping your bladder healthy:

1. **Keep hydrated:** If you have a bladder condition, there can be a strong temptation to limit the amount you drink in an effort to avoid leaks and accidents. This, however, is often counterproductive as concentrated urine, which is produced when we don't drink enough, can irritate the bladder lining. On the other hand, drinking far too much liquid can disrupt the balance of substances in our bodies such as sodium and potassium that are important for bodily function. Therefore, the key is to hydrate slowly throughout the day. For men, this should be around 2.5 litres a day (10 glasses) and for women 2 litres (eight glasses), preferably of water. However, rather than downing four glasses in the morning than another four later in the day, sip continually throughout the day (see Chapters 10 and 11). If nocturia is a problem for you (needing to get up to go to the toilet in the night), it's okay to kerb fluid intake later in the day, but do check that your urine (wee) isn't becoming too strong – there is natural variation between us all but a pale yellow colour is a sign of good hydration. Darker, strong-smelling wee can be a

sign of dehydration whereas very clear urine that looks like water may mean you're drinking too much, too quickly.

2. **Keep your pelvic floor in shape:** The results of research trials looking at how pelvic floor muscles (page 24) can help tackle incontinence consistently show that these exercises are key to taking back control over our bladders. Because this set of muscles isn't something we can see, it can be hard at first to know if we're doing the exercises correctly, and secondly to know if the muscles are becoming toned. But these simple contractions can mean that people with bladder issues can avoid medications and surgery – both of which come with risks and side effects. The exercises are very easy to do – next time you go to the toilet try to slow or stop the flow of urine and you'll be able to feel them working (but don't do this too often as disturbing your flow can eventually damage the bladder). Then (when not on the toilet) practise squeezing these muscles on a regular basis (see Chapter 9, page 101). As this exercise can be done literally anywhere, give yourself a trigger to remind you to do it; something you do many times a day such as driving or walking. Put a little note in your car or by your shoes to prompt you and after a time you'll automatically remember to practise the pelvic floor squeezing.

3. **Don't 'emergency wee':** Many of us go to the toilet 'just in case', especially people with bladder problems. However, there is an elegant mechanism that exists between the brain and bladder to let us know when it's time to find a WC and by emptying the bladder when it's not necessary, we can disrupt this process (the micturition reflex, Chapter 3, page 30). When the bladder is about half full, stretch receptors in the bladder wall tell the brain it might be a good idea to think about where a toilet is, but if there isn't one near we can hold on for quite some time – even when the bladder is over half full, we can usually manage for many hours. But if we go to the toilet many times in the day for fear

of being 'caught out', over time our bodies will think we must go to the toilet when there is very little wee to empty. Fortunately, just as going too often can mess up our bodies' understanding of when we need to urinate, we can retrain the bladder and brain back into a healthy pattern. By gradually lengthening the time between trips to the toilet or scheduling when you visit the lavatory, it's possible to once again only go when we need to go (see Chapter 9, page 99).

4. **Support your microbiota:** We are now beginning to understand how important the many millions of microorganisms in our guts are for our health. The microbiota has a vital role to play in our immune systems, so taking care of these friendly companions will help not only to keep the bladder working well, but also support overall health. This includes both physical and mental health as the gut communicates with the brain along the brain-gut axis (Chapter 4, page 37). There are many things we can do to keep the bacteria in our guts diverse, as it is the diversity of the microorganism population that seems to be key to resilience. Antibiotics are particularly damaging to the microbiota as these medicines kill off bacteria - even the good types of bacteria are affected with this treatment and can need a boost to get them back on track. You can do this by taking both pre- and probiotics as a supplement and eating foods that have pre- and probiotic properties (see Chapter 10, page 115). For people who suffer from recurrent and chronic urinary tract infections (cystitis) this is an approach worth trying. Other ways to take care of our microbiota include cutting our artificial sweeteners, cutting back on the booze, eating enough fibre and managing stress.

5. **Know your triggers:** Certain foods and drinks can trigger bladder irritation so it's useful to know which ones affect you. As different things affect different people, note down everything you eat and drink in a bladder diary. You'll

also need to write down the amount of times you needed
go to the toilet and how urgent this desire was, including
any leaks (see Chapter 10, page 115). Foods that many
people find troublesome include processed meats (it's
a good idea to avoid these anyway for general health),
some dairy products, including string cheese, cheesecakes
and flavoured yogurts, tomatoes and vegetables cooked
in tomato sauces, some fruit and spices (see Chapter 10,
page 109, for full list). Alcohol, drinks such as tea and
coffee (even the decaf versions) and fizzy drinks, including
wine, sodas and sparkling water, can also aggravate the
bladder, causing pain and urgency. To see which ones
bother you, try an exclusion diet (page 114) where all these
foods/drinks are cut out then added back into your diet
one-by-by one. Different things affect different people
and it's hard to exclude lots of foods and rinks from your
long-term diet so find out whether some of your everyday
or favourite foods are triggering symptoms.

6. **Know you're not alone:** Because bladder conditions
are embarrassing and can threaten our sense of dignity,
symptoms such as incontinence can be incredibly hard to
talk about. But bladder illness is very common indeed –
someone you know will have had bladder trouble at some
point in their lives. We are all so good at hiding health
problems that you may not even know a close friend has
experienced urgency, pain or laughter leaks. Talking about
health issues is an essential part of coping with any illness,
particularly those that are stigmatised or hidden (see
Chapter 1). Other people are not merely a shoulder to cry on
– those who have experienced the same sorts of symptoms
as us can make the world of difference, either emotionally,
practically or in terms of useful information sharing. Simply
knowing that our bodies are not so strange or unusual can
lift feelings of anxiety and despair. If you feel you can't talk

to friends or loved ones, there are many support groups for all kinds of conditions, including those covered in this book. Talking to others will also combat loneliness, which is significant for health because feeling alone is as bad for us as smoking (see below).

7. **Don't be ashamed to use products:** This doesn't just include pads and pants, although these are probably a lot better than most of us think. For light leaks, there are many options of incontinence pants that look just like regular underwear and also have odour control panels (see Chapter 15). Taking these or an extra pair of knickers or briefs with you when you're out, along with wet wipes, in a discrete toiletry bag (or a pencil case if you'd prefer) can sometimes act as a comfort crutch – even if you never use these things, you know you have them just in case. Also knowing where toilets are can help rest the mind and limit panicky feelings – there are numerous toilet locator apps and you can use a 'Just Can't Wait Card' (page 169) to ensure you don't have to stand in lengthy queues. Radar keys (page 170) allow access to over 900 accessible (and usually clean, if you do need to change clothes) toilets in the UK for people with long-term health conditions and disabilities. The important point of all these products and apps is to make sure you don't become isolated – bladder conditions are upsetting, and, for some, effective management can take time. On this journey towards recovery use everything at your disposal to continue living your life.

8. **Don't smoke and ensure you avoid other chemicals:** There is no doubt that smoking is harmful to our health. Cigarette smoke and nicotine may also irritate the bladder, leading to urgency and frequency. Smoking is the biggest risk factor for bladder cancer because the chemicals in smoking products (arylamines) pass through our bodies, eventually landing in our urine, which of course sits in

the bladder. Other chemicals (such as polycyclic aromatic hydrocarbons (PAHs)) associated with certain work, such as painting and decorating, bus and taxi driving, being a mechanic and hairdressing, are linked to bladder cancer (see Chapter 7, page 77). Hence, if you work in one of these jobs/professions and have a family history of this relatively rare cancer, try and limit other modifiable risks such as smoking. We don't yet know the long-term risks of vaping in general, let alone regarding bladder conditions (the research hasn't been done yet), so our advice is not to smoke – at all. Social support is imperative when trying to give up a habit like smoking so get your partner, family, friends and even colleagues on board with your healthy choice. Figure out your triggers for smoking too – many people smoke in an habitual pattern so jot down what you're doing when you're lighting up and work on changing these patterns with the support of loved ones.

9. **Maintain a healthy weight:** This is often easier said than done, which is why around a third of us are overweight or obese. We are constantly bombarded with food advertising, unhealthy food is around every corner and food can act as a comfort blanket. When our modern world is coupled with the fact that our bodies are evolutionarily programmed to seek out energy-dense food (usually high sugar and fat) for survival, it's not surprising that maintaining a healthy weight is challenging. But it is important when thinking about bladder health – being overweight puts a great deal of pressure on the pelvic floor muscles and bladder, leading to incontinence. Being overweight can also increase the risk of bladder cancer coming back after it has been treated (Chapter 7, page 79). Losing weight, on the other hand, can halve leaks and wetting accidents and reduce the risk of cancer recurrence, particularly in those who smoke (but try not to smoke). We often eat mindlessly throughout the day,

having little awareness of what we put into our mouths. Therefore, combine a mindful approach to eating with a diet plan full of vegetables (and some fruit, bearing in mind the sugar content) and fibre to reduce the chance of constipation.

10. **Consider your options carefully:** We all want to 'just get better' so it can be tempting to look for a quick fix. However, our bodies are complex things and so an immediate remedy rarely exists. In general, and for non-life-threatening conditions, it is best to try as many lifestyle, diet and behaviour techniques as you can before considering medications and surgical procedures. Even over-the-counter pain-killers come with side effects – for example, constipation which itself can make bladder problems worse (see Chapters 11 and 12). Aspirin and ibuprofen may also play havoc with your microbiota, reducing the numbers of good bacteria in your gut. There is always the risk of infection with surgical techniques, amongst other complications, such as water retention and pain / soreness. We've covered medications and procedures in some detail in this book because having this information allows you to make an informed choice regarding your healthcare options, but in every condition we have studied (and experienced) we've always found that, if possible, it's best to start with the things you can do yourself and which are not invasive. Sometimes medical techniques that appear well-tolerated later turn out to be harmful, so it's best to err on the side of caution and always consider your options, medical and non-medical, carefully. While the latter may take more effort, they can often be the most sustainable and risk-free methods.

Index

What's Up With Your Gut?
Why you bloat after eating bread and pasta... and other gut problems

By Jo Waters and Professor Julian Walters

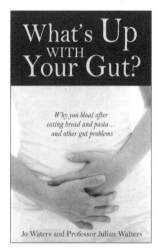

As the authors of *What's Up With Your Bladder?* describe, the essential relationship between the micro-organisms in the gut, gut function and bladder health is only now being recognised. If you have problems with your bladder you are highly likely also to have problems with your gut, so... *What's Up With Your Gut?* could give you the answers you need to start to get back to health.

www.hammersmithbooks.co.uk/product/your-gut/

Beat Chronic Disease
The nutrition solution: use functional nutrition to recover your health

By Fleur Brown

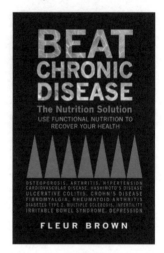

Fleur Brown, Functional Nutritionist for nearly 25 years, shares her experience of helping thousands of clients with chronic, complex health problems recover their health, vitality and well-being. She shows you how to:

- Become your own health detective to investigate the root causes of your problems
- Take charge of your health holistically
- Take steps to regain your well-being and live a full life without pain or excessive fatigue.
- Use her charts, tables and questionnaires to help yourself to better health.

www.hammersmithbooks.co.uk/product/beat-chronic-disease-nutrition-solution/

From the Nature Cures Pocktebooks series:
Recovery from Injury, Surgery and Infection

By *Nat H Hawes*

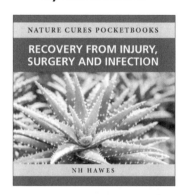

When recovering from a major health event, such as an infection or an accident or elective surgery, what you eat and drink to give your body its best chance is fundamental yet rarely discussed in mainstream medicine. This Nature Cures guide gives you the best micro- and macro-nutrients, the best herbal remedies, and the best ways to consume what you need as deliciously and effortlessly as possible.

www.hammersmithbooks.co.uk/product/recovery-from-injury/

Selected by the Reading Agency for the Reading Well scheme 2017

Irritable Bowel Syndrome
navigating your way to recovery

By Dr Megan Arroll and Professor Christine Dancey

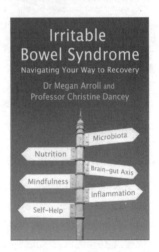

The authors of *What's Up With Your Bladder?* explore the latest research and clinical experience relating to IBS to provide an evidence-based guide to causes, diagnosis and treatment. With the authors' personal experience of invisible disease and IBS specifically (Professor Dancey co-founded the IBS Network only to discover years later that her actual problem was endometriosis), this book can make a real difference.

www.hammersmithbooks.co.uk/product/irritable-bowel-syndrome/